Foundations of Sports Coaching

Athletes and sports people at all levels rely on their coaches for advice, guidance and support. *Foundations of Sports Coaching* is a comprehensive introduction to the practical, vocational and scientific principles that underpin the sports coaching process. It provides the student of sports coaching with all the skills, knowledge and scientific background they will need to prepare athletes and sports people technically, tactically, physically and mentally. With practical coaching tips, techniques and tactics highlighted throughout, the book covers all the key components of a foundation course in sports coaching, including:

- the development of sports coaching as a profession
- coaching styles and technique
- planning and management
- basic principles of anatomy, physiology, biomechanics and psychology
- fundamentals of training and fitness
- performance analysis
- reflective practice in coaching.

Including international case studies throughout and examples from top-level sport in every chapter, *Foundations of Sports Coaching* helps to bridge the gap between coaching theory and practice. This book is essential reading for all students of sports coaching and for any practising sports coach looking to develop and extend their coaching expertise.

Paul E. Robinson is Senior Lecturer in Sports Coaching Science at the University of Chichester. He is an England Hockey Level 3 coach and a coach educator, tutor and assessor. His research interests lie in skill acquisition, specifically implicit and explicit learning and decision making.

To Victoria, Natasha, Renée and Louie

Foundations of Sports Coaching

Paul E. Robinson

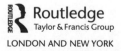 Routledge
Taylor & Francis Group

LONDON AND NEW YORK

First published 2010
by Routledge
2 Park Square, Milton Park, Abingdon, Oxon, OX14 4RN

Simultaneously published in the USA and Canada by Routledge
711 Third Avenue, New York, NY 10017

Routledge is an imprint of the Taylor & Francis Group, an Informa business

© 2010 Paul E. Robinson

Typeset in Goudy by Pindar NZ, Auckland, New Zealand
Printed and bound in Great Britain by TJ International Ltd, Padstow, Cornwall

British Library Cataloguing in Publication Data
A catalogue record for this book is available from the British Library

Library of Congress Cataloging-in-Publication Data
Robinson, Paul E.
Foundations of sports coaching / Paul E. Robinson.
    p. cm.
  Includes bibliographical references and index.
  1. Coaching (Athletics) 2. Coaches (Athletics)—Training of. I. Title.
  GV711.R63 2008
  796.07'7—dc22   2008027288

ISBN 978-0-415-46972-2 pbk
ISBN 978-0-415-46971-5 hbk
ISBN 978-0-203-88552-9 ebk

ISBN 0-415-46972-4 pbk
ISBN 0-415-46971-6 hbk
ISBN 0-203-88552-X ebk

Contents

Illustrations

FIGURES

TABLES

PHOTOS

Case studies

Preface

The reason I have chosen to write this text is to attempt to bridge the gap between coaching science and coaching practice. In sitting between the academic and vocational camps, this text will meet the particular needs of the fast growing number of students taking Foundation degrees in Sports Coaching in the UK. Hopefully the book will also appeal to those students studying on A Level, or BTEC programmes who have an interest in coaching, and to those studying on coaching related degree programmes, in order to further support their learning. I would also like to think that this text would be a source of reference to the already practising coach, who may wish to further enhance or develop their knowledge base. Although providing a mainly UK perspective on coaching, the book also looks briefly at coaching practice in Europe, North America, Australia and New Zealand. I hope by including an international perspective this will broaden the horizons of the reader, demonstrating that coaching takes place on a global scale, and that there is a lot we can learn from coaches of other nations. Equally, it is hoped that in reading this text European, American and Commonwealth coaches will gain an insight into the way coaching has developed, and is continuing to develop, here in the UK.

The nature of coaching and coaching practice is evolving, and a more informed coach is now required to support the performer. The more informed coach is one that can draw on theoretical and scientific principles, and apply them to their day-to-day coaching practice. As a practising coach and academic I have always viewed the theoretical principles that support the coaching process as "tools in a toolbox" – you pick out a tool to do the job. I know this can be seen perhaps as rather a mechanistic and simplistic view, but the successful coach cannot apply all the principles all of the time. It is important to know which tool is relevant and when. So in this context a further aim of writing this book is to provide you the coach with a range of tools with which to carry out coaching practice.

Coach education is forming a significant part in the development of coaches here in the UK, and from my research into other countries' coaching structures the same ethos seems to be applied. Considering this, it is hoped that industry professionals and Governing Bodies of Sport will find this book useful in referring to their coaching and coach education workforce, in order to support delivery of their coach education programmes.

A distinctive aspect of this text is that case studies are included from a range of coaches, development officers and volunteers in a range of sports. The rationale behind inclusion of these case studies is that it provides the student with a real-life perspective of the experiences of these individuals. With these experiences come the stresses, strains and pitfalls of sports coaching, not forgetting the feeling of elation when a coach experiences success. All of the case studies are of professionals who are currently coaching, volunteering and active in sports development in their respective sports.

With all the above in mind it is hoped that this text will be of considerable use to the reader throughout their chosen programme of study, their coaching practice and beyond into their coaching career.

Paul Robinson

Acknowledgements

I would like to thank England Hockey and especially Anne Baker, England Hockey National Coach Development Manager, for their kind permission to use material produced for England Hockey's coach education programmes. I would also like to thank the following for their time and input in developing insightful case studies: Sue Perry, a good friend and fellow coach (coaching philosophy); Louise Riddle (the role of a Sports Development Officer); Jamie Stewart-McDonald (career development in rugby); Ian Coleman (coaching high performance athletes in canoeing); Steve Fitzsimons (coaching in a basketball high performance environment); Jordan Leatherdale (how a soccer coach plans coaching sessions); Jane Lomax (how a netball coach plans her coaching sessions); Tim Holder (how a sports psychologist works with coaches); Paul Wallis (on how a fitness trainer designs and implements fitness training programmes); and Mark Scarth, SportsCoachUK South East Area Manager (career development as a coach educator).

Further thanks go to Chris Marsden (Coaching Consultant) for his continued support; Andy Gair at SportsCoachUK for his time taken to explain the process and role of the coach licensing scheme; Mark Borgers in Holland for providing information on how the Netherlands develops coaches; Mel Day for her expert coaching knowledge of trampolining which helped me construct a block planner and consider the technical requirements of another sport; Marcus Smith for his expert knowledge on boxing; Richard Clements and Simon Northcott for simplifying the section on energy systems; Danny Kerry, Great Britain women's hockey team head coach; colleagues in the Faculty of Sport, Education and Social Sciences at University of Chichester; and the Sports Coaching Science students who kindly modelled for the photographs. I would also like to thank Richard Ottaway who has been a good friend through thick and thin for over 40 years.

Finally, and by no means least, I would like to thank Simon Whitmore, Commissioning Editor, Sport and Leisure at Routledge for his valued advice, patience and support throughout this project.

All photographs courtesy of Nicola Norris (http://www.nicolanorris.co.uk).

Abbreviations

ACEP	American Coach Education Programme
ASC	Australian Sports Commission
ASEP	American Sports Education Programme
ATP	Adenosine tri-phosphate
BA	Bachelor of Arts
BASES	British Association of Sport and Exercise Sciences
BISC	British Institute of Sports Coaches
BPS	British Psychological Society
BTEC	Business and Technology Education Council
CA	Cognitive anxiety
CAC	Canadian Association of Coaches
CBAS	Coach Behaviour Assessment System
CDO	Coach Development Officer
CNS	Central nervous system
CoG	Centre of gravity
CPD	Continuing professional development
CP	Competition period
CPSU	Child Protection in Sport Unit
CRB	Criminal Record Bureau
CrP	Creatine phosphate
CRT	Choice reaction time
CSAI-2	Competitive Sport Anxiety Inventory-2
CSC	Community Sports Coach
CTS	Certificate in Tutoring Sport
DCMS	Department of Culture, Media and Sport
DFB	German Sports Council
DOMS	Delayed onset of muscle soreness
DVD	Digital Versatile Disc
EIS	English Institute of Sport
EOP	Emergency operating procedures
FA	Football Association
FE	Further Education
FIH	Federale Internationale Hockey
GB	Great Britain
GBoS	Governing Body/Bodies of Sport
GPP	General preparation period

GPS	Global Positioning System
HE	Higher Education
HPC	Health Professions Council
HPU	High Performance Unit
HUD	Heads Up Display
IAAF	International Association of Athletics Federations
IAPS	Independent Assessment Practice in Sport
ICCE	International Council for Coach Education
IOC	International Olympic Committee
KP	Knowledge of performance
KR	Knowledge of results
LTAD	Long Term Athlete Development Programme
LTM	Long-term memory
MOS	Minimum operating standards
NASC	National Association of Sports Coaches
NCAA	National College Athletic Association
NCC	National Coaching Council
NCCP	National Coaching Certification Program
NCF	National Coaching Foundation
NFHS	National Federation of State High Schools
NGB	National Governing Body
NHSCA	National High School Coaches Association
NOC*NSF	National Olympic Committee/National Sports Federation
NOP	Normal operating procedures
NSPCC	National Society of Prevention of Cruelty to Children
OBLA	Onset blood lactate accumulation
PE	Physical Education
PNS	Peripheral nervous system
PRP	Psychological refractory period
SA	Somatic anxiety
SAQ®	Speed, Agility and Quickness
SDO	Sports Development Officer
SPARC	Sport and Recreation New Zealand
SPP	Specific preparation period
SPORT	Specificity, Progression, Overload, Reversibility, Tedium
SRT	Simple reaction time
SS	Sensory store
STEPS	Space, Task, Equipment, Position, Speed
STM	Short-term memory
SWOT	Strengths, Weaknesses, Opportunities, Threats
TAIS	Test of Attentional and Interpersonal Style
TQM	Total quality management
TRP	Transition recovery period
UKCC	United Kingdom Coaching Certificate
UK	United Kingdom
USOC	United States Olympic Committee
WADA	World Anti-Doping Agency

Permissions

1. Table 2.1 is adapted with kind permission from Townend, R. and North, J. (2007). *Sports Coaching in the UK II: Main Report 2007*. SportsCoachUK, Leeds.
2. Figure 3.1 is adapted with kind permission from Lyle, J. (2002). *Sports Coaching: A Framework for Coaches' Behaviour* (Figure 3.5, p. 53). Routledge, London.
3. Figure 10.1 is adapted with kind permission from Bartlett, R. (1997). *Introduction to Sports Biomechanics* (Figure 1.9, p. 16). E & FN Spon, London.
4. Figures 10.2a and 10.2b are adapted with kind permission from Bartlett, R. (1997). *Introduction to Sports Biomechanics* (Figure 1.15a, p. 30 and Figure 1.15b, p. 31), E & FN Spon, London.
5. England Hockey kindly gave their permission for me to use material from Level 1, 2 and 3 coach education resources.

Figures 3.2, 4.1, and all figures in Chapter 5 author's own.

Introduction

There has been a significant growth of coaching related courses in a range of institutions in the UK during recent years, and at the same time a significant growth in coaching opportunities and employment, with more and more sports clubs, schools and organizations now requiring the services of a coach. Coaching will take on more significance with the 2012 London Olympics not far away and the need for coaches to support the athletes in their quest for gold. Moreover, SportsCoachUK are striving to professionalize coaching, and are implementing the UK Coaching Framework, which has a "vision of a cohesive, ethical, inclusive and valued coaching system where: skilled coaches support children, players and athletes at all stages of their development in sport, and which is number one in the world by 2016" (SportsCoachUK, 2007, p. 2).

The UK Government wants to see 50 per cent of 18–30 year olds being provided an opportunity to go into Higher Education by 2010. To achieve this, the UK Government have developed a Widening Participation initiative that creates a route into Higher Education for those who traditionally might not have thought of going to university, and they envisage Foundation degrees to be a key component in achieving that target (Halsall, 2006). With over 40 Further Education and Higher Education institutions now taking up delivering Foundation degrees in Sports Coaching or coaching related areas, and more than 150 Higher Education courses in sports coaching listed on the Education UK website, at 52 different institutions (British Council, 2008) and SportsCoachUK playing a key role in developing a world-class coaching system, there has never been a more exciting and important time to take the step into the study of sports coaching, and train to become a sports coach.

As a practising coach, coach educator and academic, this author has seen a major shift in the emphasis towards coaching in schools, clubs and in Further and Higher Education. Significant positive steps have been made to improve the standard of coaching in the UK, with GBoS having the courses they deliver being quality assured, and standardized against a specific set of criteria. Also, many sports are aligning their coaching qualifications against the United Kingdom Coaching Certificate endorsement criteria, which is a positive move forward.

A further consideration for coaching practice is continuing professional development (CPD). Coaching is an ongoing learning process, and thinking changes, as do techniques and tactics in each sport. Therefore it is important that coaches attend short courses that are delivered by a host of agencies, for example, SportsCoachUK, GBoS and UK Sport. In addition, it is essential that the practising coach in the UK has public liability insurance, a current Criminal Record Bureau check, a current first aid qualification and regularly attends child protection courses.

This book is separated into six parts, each of which begins with an introduction, outlining the content of that part. Part 1 explores sports coaching today in terms of coaching and performance, including the development of coaching. Part 1 also outlines the evolving nature of SportsCoachUK as well as providing an international perspective on sports coaching structures. Career development, coaching and the law, legal issues, coach insurance, the importance of having appropriate qualifications, the UKCC and the professionalizing of coaching are also introduced. The volunteer could be considered the backbone of British sport, and the role of the volunteer coach is explored, as is the role of Sports Development Officer in supporting the coach.

Part 2 looks at effective sports coaching. What is an effective sports coach and how does the coach become an effective coach? Part 2 introduces the skills, qualities, roles and responsibilities of a coach and the Code of Conduct for Sports Coaches both from a UK and international perspective. Part 2 also outlines and examines coaching concepts such as coaching behaviour, coaching styles, learning styles, observation and feedback. It also looks at coaching practice in terms of the processes involved in actually delivering a session from introduction to reflect and review. In addition, Part 2 highlights the fundamental principles in structuring and running practices.

Part 3 outlines the planning process and investigates the role of the coach as a manager. Many coaches when starting out will find that they are working in isolation, fulfilling a multitude of roles, such as a coach, manager, scientist, administrator, etc. It is not until they reach the higher echelons of their profession that they may have support staff working with them. Considering this, the managing of performers, teams, or squads brings its own set of challenges. A further aspect of this part of the book is season planning, which explores how the coach plans their season around the technical, tactical, physical and psychological demands of the sport being coached.

Part 4 introduces basic physiology and includes the structure and function of the skeleton, muscles, heart, lungs and digestive system. A significant section of this part of the book addresses the fundamentals of training and fitness, and the role of the coach in developing fitness programmes. Injury prevention also forms a distinctive feature of this part of the book, looking at warming up and cooling down, the warm-up decrement and the nature of injury.

A focus of Part 5 is on the psychological principles that underpin coaching practice and includes concepts such as motivation, confidence enhancement, concentration strategies and the development of pre-competition routines. Skill acquisition is also explored in detail, as the coach should have a good understanding of the processes involved in how the athlete acquires skill. A further focus in Part 5 is the coach's role in performance analysis. It is crucial that the coach has at least a basic understanding of biomechanics; therefore Part 5 will broadly outline the principles of motion, linear and angular kinematics and linear and angular kinetics, and provide some sporting practical examples. Performance analysis is a major part of the coach's "toolbox", and use of basic software packages and technology that can help support the coaching process are also highlighted.

Part 6, the final part of the book, introduces further considerations for the coach, such as coach education, coach mentoring and coaching special populations (children and disabled performers). This chapter will also highlight child protection issues and the role of the coach. The Long Term Athlete Development Programme, Lifestyle management, drugs and supplementation and the role of the coach are also explored, as is talent identification and talent transfer. Included at the end of each chapter is a seminar or discussion question designed to support the student on coach education programmes, key terms and definitions, as well as web links and a further reading list so the student can further access information.

Part 1

Sports coaching today

INTRODUCTION

This part of the book introduces a broad and contemporary view of sports coaching in the UK, coupled with brief examples of international coaching structures. Chapter 1 examines the development of coaching from a broad historical perspective in the UK, and aims to outline the emergence, role and structure of SportsCoachUK, the deployment of Coach Development Officers (Coaching Consultants) and Community Sports Coaches and the implementation and development of the UK Coaching Framework. An explanation is given of the development of the United Kingdom Coaching Certificate, and the possibility of introducing a coach licensing scheme in the UK.

Chapter 1 also provides an international perspective of coaching structures that exist in North America, Europe, Australia and New Zealand. Career development is an integral feature of this chapter, with a case study of an elite rugby player who has played for the New Zealand Divisional XV and who progressed to coaching while in NZ before becoming a head coach for a regional rugby squad in the UK that was promoted to the National League Three South Division during his tenure. Chapter 1 includes coaching and the law, in terms of litigation, negligence, legal and contractual issues; having sufficient insurance cover; and having appropriate qualifications commensurate with the level at which the coach is working. Chapter 1 also highlights how coaching is now being promoted as a profession and the issues surrounding professionalizing coaching.

Chapter 2 looks at the general role of the volunteer and the volunteer coach, who still serves as a backbone supporting sport in this country. Chapter 2 also looks at the transition from volunteer to professional coach, in terms of a reflective case study. The role of the Sports Development Officer (SDO) is also examined, supported by a case study of an existing SDO who is currently employed by a GBoS.

Chapter 3 examines coaching and performance, in particular the role of the coach working with the high performance athlete, and the chapter also looks at the differences between participation coaching and high performance coaching. At the end of each chapter suggested seminar or discussion questions are provided, along with key terms and definitions. Web links and suggested further readings are also provided if more information or further research is required.

Chapter 1

The development of coaching

CHAPTER OBJECTIVES

- Introduce a brief historical perspective on the development of coaching in the UK.
- Outline the emergence of SportsCoachUK.
- Outline coach licensing.
- Highlight the importance of having appropriate qualifications and insurance.
- Provide an awareness of the law and sports coaching.
- Highlight the importance of the UK Coaching Certificate.
- Provide an international perspective on coaching structures.
- Highlight the potential of career development in sports coaching.
- Provide a case study of a performer who has progressed into coaching.

A BRIEF HISTORICAL PERSPECTIVE

Coaching can be traced as far back as Ancient Greece, when wrestlers were instructed in the art of wrestling along with many other disciplines, which are similar to events in today's modern Olympiads. Between the fourth and fifth century BC the Greek athletes' training and preparation was a direct result of the physical education system and the special preparation for Olympic competition (Mechikoff and Estes, 1998). In Roman times ex-gladiators acted as instructors (*doctores*) and provided training in the fighting techniques and weapons of specific gladiator roles (Watkins, 1997).

In medieval Britain longbow training was mandatory and government edicts such as King Edward I's ban on sports on Sunday was designed to ensure that his people practised archery (Hickman, 2008). Formal instruction (coaching) was provided, and traditionally training began at seven years of age. McNab (1990 cited in Lyle, 2002) describes how coaching developed from the sporadic preparation of boxers and runners in the 1800s through to the early coaches of team sports in public schools, who were generally ex-university athletes who had moved into teaching.

Generally, this is how the development of coaching remained during late nineteenth to early twentieth century. During the 1930s it was realized that other countries were beginning to implement coaching structures, and coaching courses in the UK began to appear as early as then in soccer, when Stanley Rous developed the first official coaching course to be run by FA staff (Barber, 2008). However, up to the 1940s little else changed in the development of coaching. It was not until the 1950s that coach education on a national basis began to emerge (Lyle, 2002).

Cricket developed their first coaching course in 1952 (Matthews, 2008), and in 1956 the National Association of Archery Coaches developed coaching qualifications (Hodkinson, 2008). During the mid-twentieth century a strong relationship evolved between the PE teacher and sports coaching (Lyle, 2002). This relationship in part resulted in sports coaching being an extension of the role of the physical educator in schools, who were responsible for the delivery of sport in schools and supporting sport and the performer in after-school and weekend fixtures and competitions. However, this has begun to change over recent years, and there has been a shift towards providing structured coaching across a range of sports delivered by coaching professionals and PE teachers who are attending coaching-related courses and training events.

Sport England has initiated a scheme called the School Sports Programme, which aims to increase sport participation levels in primary and secondary schools (Active Schools, 2008). Coaching for teachers is part of the Schools Sport Programme and has continued to grow in strength. Over 35,000 teachers have attended courses to help them to up-skill and gain qualifications. A range of sports and activities are included in the programme, and in addition sports for young people with disabilities, support courses in first aid, umpiring and refereeing. The Coaching for Teachers programme is designed to give school teachers the skills they need to run out-of-school-hours sports activities and clubs (Active Schools, 2008).

Recently there has been another major shift towards Coach Award Courses being quality assured, aligning coaching qualifications with an awarding body, coach education, the importance of having appropriate qualifications and coaching related continual professional development. These latest developments have made significant contributions to the standard of coaching in the UK. Coaches are now becoming more informed coaches, and are embracing a range of concepts (i.e. sports science) to further develop their coaching knowledge base.

THE EMERGENCE OF SportsCoachUK

In the early 1980s the National Coaching Foundation was established in Leeds to look after the interests of coaching and coaches (SportsCoachUK, 2008a).

This organization was supported by a range of sporting bodies in British sport and was formed to establish a comprehensive non-specific sport coach education programme throughout the United Kingdom catering for all levels of coach. A series of key events from 1986 through to 2001 has seen the National Coaching Foundation evolve into SportsCoachUK, and these are summarized below (further detail can be found on the SportsCoachUK website under "About Us" in "Our History").

In 1986 a focus group was established with a remit to produce a coaching strategy for the future. In 1987 a network of 14 National Coaching Centres was established that designated the Coaching Arm of the (Great Britain) Sports Council with responsibility for the coordination of coaching and coach education. In 1988 the Sports Council reported that it regarded the implementation of the National Coaching Foundation, and network of National Coaching Centres throughout the UK, as one of the major successes of the past five years (Sports Council, 1988) cited in (SportsCoachUK, 2008a). In 1990 independence was gained from the (GB) Sports Council, and a trading subsidiary was established, known as Coachwise Ltd. The Champion Coaching scheme was created, establishing a range of coaching initiatives led by GBoS to provide coaching for children. In 1993 a membership service was formed which gave advice and guidance on product development and services. By 1995 the Champion Coaching initiative was providing quality coaching for thousands of young people in over a hundred schemes, which involved over 300 coaches.

In 1997, 18,000 coaches took advantage of the wide range of professional opportunities available at national, regional and local levels and the Australian Coaching Council made a request to use elements of the NCF coach education programme themselves to develop a coach education programme in Australia (SportsCoachUK, 2008a). In 1999 Coaching for Teachers provided over 800 courses attended by over 12,000 teachers and a new workshop programme was launched in January 1999. Also, Premier Coaching Centres were established in strategically placed locations that allowed coaches access to a range of courses, products and resources. *Faster, Higher, Stronger* (now *Coaching Edge*), the UK's quarterly magazine for coaching, and the High Performance coaching programme were launched.

In 2000 NCF membership services were launched and over 2,500 development opportunities were provided by the NCF, attended by over 30,000 coaches and teachers (SportsCoachUK, 2008a). In 2001 the NCF was re-branded as SportsCoachUK, and 1st4sport Qualifications, a new awarding body meeting the criteria set by the Qualifications and Curriculum Authority was established as a trading division within Coachwise.

In 2002 *The Coaching Task Force Final Report* (DCMS, 2002) was produced by the Department of Culture, Media and Sport, Sport and Recreation Division, and was wide-ranging in its scope, context and recommendations. The report identified a need for an investment in coaching and consistent coach development, and suggested that coach education should be a focus. It also recommended that future coach deployment and employment should also be considered. The full report can be accessed on the DCMS website (see web link at the end of this chapter).

Subsequently, in 2004 (facilitated by Sport England and SportsCoachUK), 30 Coach Development Officers (CDOs) were appointed, whose main purpose was to work with the emerging County Sports Partnerships, GBoS, schools, FE/HE institutes, local authorities and other key stakeholders to support the sustainable implementation of continuous professional development for identified coaches (SportsCoachUK, 2008b). By 2006 a further 15 CDOs were appointed, bringing the workforce up to 45. To support these CDOs, eight Regional Coaching Managers were appointed to oversee the work of the CDOs, who were divided over the eight UK regions.

A further recommendation of *The Coaching Task Force Final Report* (2002) was to provide more opportunities for coaches to develop coaching as a career. In response to this, Sport England, funded by the DCMS, established the Community Sports Coach scheme. The objective of this scheme was to establish 3,000 paid qualified Community Sports Coaches (CSCs) working at a local level to increase the number and range of coaching opportunities according to strategic and local need by 2006 (Green, 2003). This scheme has been a great success, with many people gaining opportunities in coaching employment.

In 2005 SportsCoachUK began developing the UK Action Plan for Coaching in partnership with GBoS and the key funding agencies: UK Sport, the Department for Culture, Media and Sport, the Home Country Sports Councils, the Department for Education and Skills, the British Olympic Association, Youth Sport Trust and Skills Active. In 2006 a wide-ranging process of consultation was undertaken which spanned all of that year and some way into 2007, the findings of which resulted in development and implementation of the UK Coaching Framework, which identifies clear targets to further enhance coaching in the UK (SportsCoachUK, 2008d). In July 2006 calls for proposals to host the UK Centre for

Coaching Excellence in sport and disability sport were promulgated, and in June 2008 it was announced that this centre would be based at Leeds Metropolitan University.

In 2007 the UK Coaching Framework was officially launched at the 3rd UK Coaching Summit in Coventry in April 2008. In early 2008 SportsCoachUK went through a strategic review, one result of which was that the CDOs' roles were re-aligned and they became Coaching Consultants. In May 2008, the Government made a significant commitment to improving skills by giving the go-ahead on a National Skills Academy for Sport and Active Leisure that would focus on improving the standard of training of coaches across England and thereby give athletes training towards the 2012 Olympics an even better chance of claiming a place on the medals podium (SportsCoachUK, 2008i). In 2009 the 4th UK Coaching Summit was held in Glasgow, and the UK Coaching Framework transited from the "foundation" stage to the "delivering the goals" stage (Duffy, 2009).

SportsCoachUK and GBoS are now taking more of a lead in developing and implementing coaching policy. The UK Coaching Framework is an example of a coaching policy that has been developed and is being implemented in stages, with many GBoS taking the principles of the framework onboard. SportsCoachUK, along with GBoS, is a major organization supporting coaching and coaches in the United Kingdom, offering a range of services to facilitate this. These include workshops, learning resources, a quarterly magazine, coaching information, employment opportunities and research information.

SportsCoachUK is also making big strides in ensuring that coaching becomes a recognized profession, and are investigating moving towards a coach licensing scheme which some GBoS are supporting and are already beginning to implement.

COACH LICENSING

SportsCoachUK is investigating whether a need exists to develop and implement a coach licensing scheme for the sports coach. Sports such as tennis and athletics have introduced schemes as part of their Coach Awards and with the introduction and development of UKCC endorsed coaching qualifications, other sports are also considering following suit (SportsCoachUK, 2008h). SportsCoachUK has begun a consultation process and is exploring the possibilities of developing such a scheme UK-wide.

It is also investigating what quality standards would be required to ensure parity in licensing exists across all sports who express an interest in implementing the scheme. In essence it will mean that certain criteria will have to be met (i.e. appropriate qualifications for the ability you are coaching, being insured, etc.) in order for the coach to practice. This is a positive move forward and will further serve to professionalize coaching and create a regulated and quality assured coaching culture.

APPROPRIATE QUALIFICATIONS AND INSURANCE

The practising coach should always have appropriate and current insurance, and they should also have qualifications that are commensurate with the ability they are coaching. Unfortunately, in a range of sports there are still individuals who have no coaching qualification and still operate as coaches. Moreover, there are others who tout themselves as a higher-level coach than they actually are. As well as being unethical, there are massive implications if anything goes wrong.

Unfortunately, we live in a litigious society and the potential for being taken to court for negligence is omnipresent. If the coach does not have the appropriate qualification to match the task and ability he or she is delivering and does not have appropriate insurance cover, then they could find themselves involved in a lengthy, complicated and unnecessary court case. For as little as £40 (at the time of going to press) insurance is available which covers the coach for up to £5 million public liability indemnity.

COACHING AND THE LAW

Modern life is permeated and supported by a range of different legal frameworks which impact upon our work and leisure time, and the sports coach is not exempt from this. Coaches need to be aware of how the law of the land can affect coaching, and awareness needs to be raised because recently there has arisen a culture of public litigation which has spawned a generation of no-win, no-fee lawyers (Gardner, 1999). This has been coupled with a step change in social attitudes towards sport and to some extent the media exposure of bad practice (SportsCoachUK, 2008e).

In 2004 The FA was being sued for up to £700,000 in compensation by its former coach Les Reed, who was an assistant under-21s coach, claiming that he was sacked without notice (Newman, 2004). In 2000 two Canadian coaches were involved in a lawsuit with claims levelled against them on team selection issues (Centre for Sport and Law, 2000). In 2009 a women's basketball coach in Michigan, USA was in the process of being sued by a former player, who claimed her heterosexuality was a factor in losing a scholarship (AP, 2009).

Four sources of liability have been identified that may directly apply to coaching and coaching practice: negligence, contract and employment, statutes and disciplinary issues (Gardner, 1999). Negligence relates to your duty of care towards an athlete; violating a standard; infringement of organization or institutional rules; loss, harm, damage or injury to the performer; or dereliction of duty that contributes to the harm or loss of the athlete (SportsCoachUK, 2008e).

For many years the issue of contracts for coaches did not exist – only a verbal gentlemen's agreement determined the coach's roles and responsibilities working at a club. However, it is advisable that even if a coach is working for a club or organization at the grass roots level either on a full- or part-time basis a contractual agreement should be drawn up. This is as much to protect both parties involved in the agreement as to operate at a professional level. There are specific and necessary elements that make up a binding contract, such as an offer and acceptance, a statement setting out the intention that the contract is to be legally binding and that the supplier (the coach) will carry out the service (coaching duties as stated in the contract) with reasonable care and skill. A statement may exist where a consideration (a fee) is to be paid, and at what intervals (weekly, monthly or at the end of the contract) (SportsCoachUK, 2008e).

There are also certain statutes that the coach should be aware of, which may impinge upon their coaching practice. These include the Children Act 1989, the Race Relations Act 1976, the Sexual Discrimination Act 1976, the Equal Opportunities Act 2004 (Gardner, 1999) and the Disability Discrimination Act 1995. These statutes are also updated from time to time, and should be consulted on a regular basis in order to keep abreast of changes in legislation that may affect coaching practice.

Disciplinary issues may also apply in coaching practice and can range from constitutional and/or contractual issues; not adhering to organizational policies and procedures; abusing position; and abuse of a performer. While none of these issues are common in coaching at present, coaching practice as an industry is becoming more and more regulated and many coaching-practice issues are falling under the umbrella of employment law.

The coach will also have to consider his or her employment status, with regard to being employed by a company or institution or being self-employed. Generally, when employed by a large organization tax and national insurance will be deducted at source. If the coach is self-employed and tax and national insurance deductions are still applicable, it is the coach's responsibility to declare his/her earnings. An HM Customs and Revenue self-assessment form needs to be completed and returned each financial year outlining income and expenditure, in order that tax and national insurance contributions can be deducted.

THE UK COACHING CERTIFICATE

A further development in coaching in the United Kingdom is the implementation of the United Kingdom Coaching Certificate. The UK Coaching Certificate (UKCC) is a process by which GBoS coach education programmes are endorsed against an agreed set of criteria (SportsCoachUK, 2008c). A range of sports (for example, badminton, cricket, cycling, hockey, rugby league, squash, table tennis and netball) have been endorsed for either Level 1, Levels 1 and 2 or Levels 1, 2 and 3 and some "trail blazer" sports such as England Hockey are now working on developing the UKCC Level 4 Coach Award specific to their own sport. More sports are embracing the UKCC and aligning their coaching qualifications with the endorsement criteria.

What this means for the coach starting out in their career is that they will know that the general coaching process is standardized across a range of sports, with the obvious exception of the technical requirements of each sport being different. The UKCC has also enabled parity to be made in qualifications across a range of sports, which allows them to be transferable (this was not the case prior to the implementation of the UKCC). This now means that the length of course and the generic coaching principles and processes for a Level 1 Coach Award in for example rugby and cricket will be the same; only the technical definition will be different.

For a full and up-to-date list of all the endorsed sports and at what level they are endorsed at, access the United Kingdom Coaching Certificate website (see web link at the end of this chapter).

AN INTERNATIONAL PERSPECTIVE

An international body now exists that promotes the interests of coaches and coach education on a global scale. The International Council for Coach Education (ICCE) is an international organization with the mission of promoting coaching as an internationally accepted profession. The primary focus of the members, who are highly placed senior coaches, sport coaching policy makers and world leaders in coach development and education, is to increase the quality of coaching at every level of sport (ICCE, 2008). For further information on this organization see the web link at the end of this chapter.

During the 1970s, Rainer Martens founded the American Coaching Effectiveness Programme (ACEP), which later evolved into the American Sport Education Programme (ASEP). In 1981 the first ASEP course was produced and released, and by 1986 ASEP had 1,400 certified instructors who had trained more than 50,000 coaches (ASEP, 2008). In the early 1990s ASEP developed a series of advanced coaching courses based on sport, physiology, psychology and biomechanics (Martens, 2004). In 1990 ASEP partnered with high schools to offer versions of coaching courses, and since 2006 ASEP has worked directly with high school associations in delivering the ASEP Professional Coaches Education Programme to more than 25,000 coaches a year, and it also operates a Volunteer Coaching Education Programme (ASEP, 2008).

In the USA a coach education programme has recently been implemented by the United States Field Hockey Association providing three levels of certification, and the US National High School Coaches Association has also implemented a coaching certification programme for their members (see web link at the end of this chapter for further information).

The Canadian Association of Coaches (CAC) was established in 1970 as a result of recommendations of the Task Force on Sport for Canadians and exists to support coaches and coach development and improve coaching effectiveness across all levels of sport in Canada (CAC, 2005). In 1974, the CAC launched the National Coaching Certification Program (NCCP) and has developed into a world leader in coach training and certification. Each year, more than 50,000 coaches participate in an NCCP workshop and since it began not far short of one million coaches have participated in the programme (CAC, 2005).

In New Zealand the importance of coaching and having a world-class coaching system was recognized by the New Zealand Government. In 2001 a ministerial taskforce report summarized that coaching in New Zealand needed go through a process of comprehensive review and updating in order to evolve and keep pace with the rest of the world (SPARC, 2004).

In response to this report, in 2003 New Zealand developed the National Coaching Strategy and the High Performance Coaching Strategy, which consequently evolved into the *New Zealand Coaching Strategy: Taking Coaching into the Future* (SPARC, 2004). The strategy highlighted three objectives that must be achieved which are to "increase the quality and quantity of time available for coaches to focus on coaching and coach education opportunities, increase the recognition and status of coaches and to continually improve the quality of the coach education process" (SPARC, 2004), thereby ensuring that appropriate pathways exist for further development. New Zealand has clearly identified that high quality coaching is necessary in providing a positive influence on the lives of those who receive it. Sport and Recreation New Zealand (SPARC) have since introduced a range of policies to support the 2004 strategy. For more information access the SPARC web link at the end of this chapter.

In Australia the first step towards Australia's national approach to coaching stemmed from a 1973 report that suggested coaching at the international level should no longer be contingent on techniques and information which are passed down from the coach to the player, who then becomes a coach (ASC, 2008a). In 1975 an Australian Sports Institute report suggested that Australian coaching standards would not improve unless a structured coaching programme with a qualification framework was established. In 1978, in response to this report, the National Coaching Council (NCC) was established which implemented a National Coaching Accreditation Scheme comprised of three levels (ASC, 2008a). Two years later, in 1980, the NCC was in a position to approve coaching courses in a range of sports, and coaches began to receive their qualifications in September of that year. In 1990 the Australian Coaching Council introduced the Australian Coach Awards, which recognized the hard work and dedication that coaches devoted to sport in Australia (ASC, 2008a). For further information, access the Australian Sports Commission web link at the end of this chapter.

In Europe different organizations and structures exist that support sport and coaching. Constraints on the level of content in this text will dictate that only brief examples from a selection of countries can be provided. However, see the web link at the end of this chapter to conduct further research into European countries' sports coaching organizations and structures.

In Germany, at the federal level, the responsibility for top-level sport lies with the Federal Ministry of the Interior and it is the local authorities who are essentially involved in the

13

promotion of recreational sport. Coach education Level 1, 2 and 3 courses are administered by the DFB (German Sports Council) (Nash, 2003).

In France the Ministry of Youth and Sports and the Ministry of Education are responsible for most physical and sporting activities. The Ministry of Youth and Sports is responsible for promoting all forms of sporting activities for all age groups, for the management and supervision of State Aid support to sports groups, and for defining and implementing training schemes for voluntary or professional sports leaders (i.e. coaches) (Hughes and Reader, 2003). In 1976 the National Institute of PE and Sport was founded and is located on the outskirts of Paris. This is France's National Sports Academy, where most top athletes train and teachers and coaches are taught and developed (Hughes and Reader, 2003).

In the Netherlands the NOC*NSF (National Olympic Committee/National Sport Federation) sets the basic rules in relation to sport and coaching, and is closely connected to the different federations that each represent their own sport. In essence, the sport-specific NGBs deliver the courses but they are under some guidance from the NOC*NSF (Borgers, 2008).

CAREER DEVELOPMENT IN COACHING

Coaching is starting to emerge as a profession in its own right and will be elevated to a profession acknowledged as core to the development of sport and the individual (SportsCoachUK, 2008j). This is being helped by higher quality coaching courses being delivered by GBoS, opportunities for CPD and more opportunities for paid employment in coaching, and of course by the unstinting work of SportsCoachUK to improve standards.

There is a range of career opportunities for coaches, such as a multi-skills coach working for a local authority, working for a County Sports Partnership, becoming a generalist community sports coach or a sport-specific community sports coach. There are also coaching opportunities in schools, private hotels or leisure companies, sports clubs or GBoS (SportsCoachUK, 2008k), and gap-year volunteer coaching opportunities even exist abroad in a range of sports (see the web link at the end of this chapter). Opportunities are arising for coaches to work in schools, and Griggs (2008) highlights that a number of sports coaches are delivering sports sessions in primary school. In many schools throughout the UK after-school clubs and extra-curricular activities are being implemented and for students who are keen on sport, going into schools to run sports can be the first step to becoming a coach (Continyou, 2007).

Commercial sports coaching companies are now emerging that are offering employment to sports coaches to work in schools, and an internet search will provide information on a range of these companies. In order to access coaching courses directly, the individual should contact their GBoS to request details of their Coaching Award structure, and of dates and courses running in a particular region.

Another route into coaching is to apply to educational institutions. FE and HE institutions offer courses at different entry levels, and entry is decided on basis of ability in and commitment to sport, as well as academic ability, of course. Involvement in schools and experience of helping with activities at club level will also be advantage, and a degree in a sports related subject or in professional teaching can also be beneficial. GBoS are responsible for Coach Award delivery and coach education and one cannot progress as a sports coach without a coaching qualification in your particular sport, even if you have an academic qualification (SportsCoachUK, 2008k).

Many GBoS have clear coach development pathways identified in their Coach Award schemes, which allows for progression from grass roots to coaching in the high performance environment with elite performers. An individual can sit at any level they desire; it is not everyone's ambition to coach at the top level. Many coaches are quite happy working at the grass roots or improvers level, which is just as important as working at the top level.

The following organizations regularly advertise for coaches in paid positions: SportsCoachUK, Sport England, UK Sport, County Sports Partnerships, GBoS, Local Government Sports Development Units, sports clubs, schools and FE and HE institutions. Also, over the last five years there has been a large increase in HE institutions offering coaching-related courses. So in view of this and with the advent of the 2012 London Olympics, the coaching industry is only going to grow, and therefore the opportunities for coaching employment are only going to increase.

Case study 1.1 – Career development

Jamie is a professional rugby coach who has played for the New Zealand (NZ) Divisional XV and who progressed to coaching while in NZ and eventually became a head coach for a regional rugby squad in the UK. Jamie was also involved in teaching on a Level 2 Sports Coaching Science programme at a UK university. Jamie started playing schoolboy rugby at the age of 13 in Taranaki, NZ. Due to the school team's ability not being high enough, when Jamie reached 16 years old he joined his local club and started playing for the club under-21 side. Jamie then went on to university and soon progressed to regional representative level while enrolled in an adventure education programme at university. The following year he moved to Waikato University and studied for a BA Leisure degree and played rugby for the university side who play in the first division of the regional league. Jamie also trialled for NZ universities, but was not selected because of his involvement in other sports. An opportunity then arose with a top club side in his hometown. However, he soon found that studying and playing rugby began to compete with each other, and he decided to follow a rugby-playing career.

The following year he moved clubs in order to try and break into the National Provincial Competition (equivalent to rugby National League Division 2 in England). During this period he worked at a local gym and attended short professional development courses which enabled him to deliver strength and conditioning sessions at his rugby club. This was Jamie's first break into delivering fitness programmes and coaching. Jamie also was a member of the local Surf Life Saving Club, and delivered a variety of courses that supported Surf Life Saving. Being part of this environment was also a valuable experience in terms of developing coaching knowledge and practice. Jamie soon progressed into the 1st XV of the Wairarapa Bush (National Provincial Competition side), who were also a semi-professional side, and he played for them for three seasons. Into his third season he trialled for the NZ Divisional XV, which is a nationally recognized NZ side who play international test rugby against Pacific Island teams (e.g. Tonga, Samoa), Japan and Canada, etc. to help prepare these nations for World Cups and other major test matches.

Because of his education and work experience Jamie was increasingly asked to take more coaching sessions, which mostly consisted of strength and conditioning work, and he was influenced by many strength and conditioning trainers (including Ashley Jones and Paul Check) when attending conferences and courses. Jamie then moved clubs to Poneke Wellington and set up a rugby performance academy for young aspiring rugby players at which he was also responsible for coaching. This period was also the time that Jamie began the transition from player to player-coach, and began to enjoy both roles. During this period Jamie started to develop a coaching profile and attend formal Coach Award schemes, such as Kiwi Sport and Coaching Association of New Zealand coaching qualifications at Level 1 and Level 2. Needing a change of focus, in 2004 Jamie decided to come to the UK for an extended holiday and visited the South of England. A friend suggested that he look at a local regional rugby club as they were looking for good-level rugby players who also had coaching experience. The regional rugby club invited him to have a look at the playing and coaching set-up to see if it would suit what he was looking for in terms of playing and coaching. Seeing this as a good opportunity Jamie decided to take the chance to experience playing and coaching in another country.

At the same time Jamie enrolled at a local university as an international student choosing to study for a Sports Coaching Science degree. He also viewed this as another opportunity to gain an academic qualification in a sports-related area which would further enhance his knowledge base, and potentially further his career. In his role as development officer for the club, he has coached at a number of schools in the local region, and has had the opportunity to attend a range of courses in order to further his CPD.

Jamie has found there are differences in the way coaching is viewed, delivered and practised in the UK compared to NZ. One of the main differences is that in the UK coaching is a lot more focused on health and safety issues, and coaches have more concerns regarding litigation and the compensation culture that is becoming more prevalent. This is not to say there is lack of awareness of health and safety issues in NZ, but it seems that the litigation and compensation culture in the UK could be considered as over-bearing. A difference also exists in coaching philosophy in terms of the way certain elements or practices are delivered (less full contact is delivered in training in NZ compared to the UK). Jamie found this difficult to understand, questioning the logic of full contact in training, when there is potential for injury, and thinking it should be left to competition.

A further difference was that he initially found it difficult to adapt his coaching style to the more democratic delivery expected in the UK, in comparison to NZ where a more autocratic style was expected and delivered. In NZ, especially in rugby, there seems to be more of a competitive edge between players, and players and coach, with an attitude from the coach of "get on with it, if you don't like it – tough", and this is accepted by all the players.

Jamie's coaching aspirations on return to NZ involve moving into coach development and coach education, and ultimately delivering coaching science courses at a NZ university. In terms of his career development, a clear pathway is visible from player to player-coach, and subsequently to coach, and a range of experiences have shaped Jamie into the coach he is now. Jamie's continued philosophy as a coach is ensuring that young people progress their skills and enjoy their sport, and for elite players to develop and maximize their potential.

SUMMARY

Although sports coaching can be traced back to Ancient Greek and Roman times, it has only been during the last century, and especially since the inception of SportsCoachUK, that coaching has developed into a recognizable career path. With the development of strategies, initiatives and policies such as the UK Coaching Framework, UKCC and Coach Licensing, coaching in the UK is starting to be recognized as a profession. It is essential that the coach holds appropriate qualifications and is adequately insured in order to practise coaching. Coaching is now starting to fall under the umbrella of employment law, so it is also essential that the sports coach is knowledgeable regarding current legislation related to disability and equality issues, as well as contractual issues. It not only the UK that seems to be vigorously promoting and developing sports coaching, but other countries are also seeing the importance and benefit of having an effective coaching structure in place in order to support their athletes.

SEMINAR OR DISCUSSION QUESTIONS

1. What is the role and function of SportsCoachUK, and what purpose does the UK Coaching Framework serve?
2. Compare different countries' coaching structures.

KEY TERMS AND DEFINITIONS

■   Coach licensing – a policy that is being considered by SportsCoachUK, in order to regulate the coaching industry.
■   Department of Media, Culture and Sport – government department responsible for government policy on sport.
■   Governing Body of Sport – a sport-specific organization that looks after all the interests of that sport.
■   United Kingdom Coaching Certificate – an endorsement of coach education programmes across sports within the UK set against agreed criteria.

WEB LINKS

Australian Sports Commission – www.ausport.gov.au/
The Autonomy of Sport in Europe – www.euoffice.eurolympic.org/cms/?p=296&s=eoc_simplecontent&
Coaching employment opportunities – www.jobswithballs.com
Department of Culture, Media and Sport – www.dcms.gov.uk
European Sport Commision – http://ec.europa.eu/sport/index_en.htm
European Sport Structures – www.euoffice.eurolympic.org/cms/?p=293&s=eoc_simplecontent&
Gap-year coaching opportunities – www.unitedthroughsport.org
International Council for Coach Education – www.icce.ws/about
National High School Coaches Association – www.nhsca.com
SportsCoachUK – www.sportscoachuk.org
Sport England – www.sportengland.org
Sport and Recreation New Zealand – www.sparc.org.nz/sport/coaching/overview
United Kingdom Coaching Certificate – www.sportscoachuk.org/index.php?PageID=3&sc=9&uid=
    (Students can register through the SportsCoachUK website – www.sportscoachuk.org)
UK Sport – www.uksport.gov.uk

FURTHER READING

DCMS (2002). *The Coaching Task Force Final Report*. Sport and Recreation Division of Department of Culture, Media and Sport. UK Government, England.
Jarvie, G. (2006). *Sport, Culture and Society*. Routledge, London.
Lyle, J. (2002). *Sports Concepts: A Framework for Coaches' Behaviour*. Routledge, London.

Chapter 2

Volunteering and coaching

⚡

CHAPTER OBJECTIVES

- Examine the role of the coach as a volunteer.
- Provide a reflective case study on volunteering and coaching.
- Outline the role of the Sports Development Officer in supporting coaching.
- Provide a case study of a current Sports Development Officer working for a GBoS.

THE ROLE OF THE COACH AS A VOLUNTEER

A volunteer is defined as an individual who helps others in sport through formal organizations such as clubs or GBoS while receiving no remuneration except expenses (English Sports Council, 1996). The sports volunteer contributes a significant amount of time and effort in supporting sport in the UK. The English Sports Council 1996 summary of major findings from a Sports Council survey into the voluntary sector of UK sport estimates that the total annual value of the UK sports volunteer market is over £1.5 billion. Sport England reported in 2003 that there were over 5.8 million volunteers contributing 1.2 billion hours each year to sport and argued that without volunteer involvement sports would struggle to survive (Sport England, 2003). Among this volunteer workforce of officials, administrators, parents, helpers, etc. is the sports coach, who dedicates many hours during evenings and weekends in order to improve the performer without regard to his or her own recognition or reward.

Volunteer coaches play an important and significant role in supporting sport in the UK, and they are the backbone of many clubs and organizations. Many sports clubs and organizations, because of their amateur and volunteer status, are unable to pay for professional coaches and staff, so this core workforce of parents, helpers and volunteer coaches is crucial in the servicing of the voluntary sector.

The 2004 SportsCoachUK survey suggested that 81 per cent of coaches were unpaid (i.e. voluntary coaches), 14 per cent were part-time paid and 5 per cent were full-time paid (SportsCoachUK, 2008f). The *Sports Coaching in the UK II: Main Report 2007* (Townend and North, 2007) which followed showed that voluntary coaching had reduced, and paid coaching had shown an increase. The largest rise was seen in part-time paid coaching, with a slight increase in full-time paid coaching. Even with a major focus to professionalize and enhance the status of the coach, data show that around 69 per cent of the sports coaching workforce

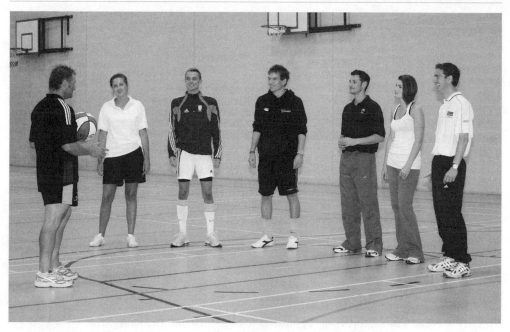

Photo 2.1 The coach addressing a group of performers.

were voluntary during this period. However, a change is again evident between 2007 and 2008. Data compiled in *The Coaching Workforce 2009–2016* report (North, 2009) shows a 6 per cent increase in the volunteer workforce, a 3 per cent decrease in part-time paid coaches and a 4 per cent drop in the number of full-time paid coaches. The percentage of the volunteers in the coaching workforce rose to 76 per cent for the 2008 period, which is sizeable.

The challenge is to convert a portion of the volunteer workforce into part-time, and a portion of the part-time into full-time paid coaches. Table 2.1 shows data from the *Sports Coaching in the UK II: Main Report 2007* and *The Coaching Workforce 2009–2016* report, and the ratios of coaches in each sector.

Voluntary coaching plays an important role in the professional development of a coach, in terms of gaining coaching experience with a range of performers in different coaching environments. However, there is an issue in terms of volunteer coaches who give up a lot of time supporting sports clubs without having formal qualifications, which may be due to them not having the time or money to attend a course, or to them being quite happy volunteering without having to go through the process of gaining formal qualifications. This does raise an issue, in terms of ensuring that everyone who coaches has the requisite qualifications and insurance cover, and has attended child protection courses. There are courses the volunteer coach can attend, however, such as the Junior Sports Leader Award, Higher Sports Leader Award and GBoS Leadership Awards prior to commencing a GBoS Level 1 Coach Award. These awards are generally delivered in schools and FE centres, and can mark the first step into the coaching profession for the young volunteer.

Clubs also play an important role in developing the volunteer and providing opportunities for young people to engage and develop into leadership roles, which may consequently provide further opportunities to develop as a coach. Sport England acknowledges and fully appreciates the hard work that is put in by sports clubs to develop and nurture high quality,

Table 2.1 *Coaches by employment type and ratios for each sector*

	Number	%	VC – FT	VC – PT	PT – FT
				Ratios	
Volunteer coach					
2007	822,000	70	10.5 to 1	3.0 to 1	3.6 to 1
2008	841,716	76	23 to 1	3.6 to 1	6.3 to 1
Part-time paid coach					
2007	277,000	24			
2008	230,765	21			
Full-time paid coach					
2007	78,000	7			
2008	36,537	3			

Source: 2007 data: Townend and North (2007); 2008 data: North (2009)

welcoming environments for young participants who aspire to take on a leadership role, and they are seen an essential part of supporting the sporting infrastructure in England (Sport England, 2002).

To support the development of sports clubs the Clubmark accreditation scheme was introduced by Sport England in 2002 to ensure that good practice and minimum operating standards (MOS) are delivered through all club development. Clubmark accreditation is awarded to clubs that comply with MOS in four areas (Clubmark, 2008). The first MOS concerns the playing programme, for example setting out guidelines for coach-to-young-person ratio, contact details of coaches at the club and which coach is allocated to a specific junior team for training and competition. The MOS of duty of care and child protection outline a range of standards to be met, for example that all coaches must have read and understood such documents as the Code of Conduct for Sports Coaches, must know what to do in an emergency when they are coaching and must have attended child protection training.

For the MOS of sports equity and ethics, the club or organization should ensure that coaches understand the policies and procedures that are set out in the organizational constitution that impact upon equity and ethical issues when coaching. Finally, for the club management criteria to be met, the club has, for example, to ensure that recruitment and selection of coaches is conducted in a fair and equitable manner, and that the club, along with the coaching structure, is sound constitutionally. For further information access the web link at the end of this chapter.

Case study 2.1 – A career reflection

In the early stages of my career I dedicated a large part of my time to volunteer coaching. I had a firm view that I should try to do as much coaching in a range of different contexts (male and female, junior and adult) as a volunteer in order to gain as much experience as possible. I also realized that during this period I should also gain formal coaching qualifications so that I could coach knowing I was appropriately qualified to deliver at the ability levels I was working with. After taking the England Hockey Level 1 Coach Award I found that other doors began to open, and more coaching work was available both voluntary and paid. This I found a valuable experience in my development as a coach. During this time I was coaching at junior club level (as an assistant coach), as well as coaching a college side and a university men's and ladies side. I then decided two years after taking my Level 1 coaching qualification to attend a Level 2 Coach Award, which I passed.

I was now a head coach in my own right, and I had three paid coaching jobs (college, university and a club team) which were all in a part-time capacity. While a Level 2 qualified coach I still carried out a lot of voluntary work, which I viewed as an important facet in my development as a coach. For four years I was head coach for Sussex County under-19 boys, which was a volunteer role. This role was time-consuming, and I travelled around the South of England at my own expense. However, it was one of my most rewarding experiences as a coach, the team having won back-to-back county championships, and I was working with a very good group of young hockey players.

During this period I set up a youth development scheme in the local district to introduce children to hockey. Local school children attended a coaching programme over an eight-week period which was in partnership with the local council sports development unit, college, university and local hockey club. This again I found very rewarding, and was done purely on a volunteer basis. This programme had the added bonus of developing young coaches and leaders who assisted in delivery of the coaching sessions. During this period I also realized the importance of continuing professional development (CPD) and attended a range of SportsCoachUK, local government sport development training courses, and GBoS short courses. I also began my coach education tutor training in order to become a registered and qualified coach educator for my GBoS. After being a Level 2 coach for five years I decided to attend the Level 3 Coach Award, which I passed.

While a Level 3 coach I continued to do some voluntary work, however, I did find that there were further demands made on me as a more highly qualified coach, which meant I had limited time to fit everything in. Therefore, I was unable to carry out as much voluntary work as I would have liked. I did however, spend just over a year with the South of England under-17 boys' squad, which was a voluntary post at the time, and again this was a rewarding and valuable experience.

By now I was a full-time, paid professional coach working in a range of scenarios, with a range of abilities, ages and genders, and this along with a full-time job. Even as a Level 3 coach, I continued with my CPD and attended a range of short courses, which further developed me as a coach. It has only been more recently that I have not carried out any voluntary work, which is due to time constraints, but I still continue to attend CPD events and courses. The only coaching I do now is for the local university men's side, and I am still involved with coach education for my GBoS, delivering Coach Awards and assessing coaches on their practical delivery for their final coaching assessments. I also have written coach education resources for my GBoS.

My philosophy now is to pass on my knowledge and experience to up-and-coming coaches and develop them in the hope that they also have the same positive experiences as my self. The main points that are raised through my own personal experience of going through the transition from player to coach and volunteer to professional coach is that volunteer coaching is an important part of any coach's development. Also, there is the opportunity to work alongside other experienced coaches in order to learn your "trade". Another of my reasons for doing so much volunteer coaching was to give back what my sport had given me over a period of years. In many ways I was a lot happier with not being paid than I was being paid as a coach – unfortunately being paid does bring its own problems at times. Also, as a volunteer, many CPD opportunities arose through the organizations I was coaching for, which I was encouraged to take. This again was an important part of my development as a coach, and I learnt a lot from other areas that impact upon coaching practice, plus a range of networks opened up for me in order to further support my coaching. In essence it is highly recommended that any coach who is starting out on his or her career at least does some volunteer coaching in order to develop themselves; it is a rewarding experience.

THE ROLE OF A SPORTS DEVELOPMENT OFFICER IN SUPPORTING COACHING

Sports coaches require a sustained support network: this is regardless of whether the coach is a volunteer or a professionally paid coach. One of these sources of support is the Sports Development Officer (SDO). The role of a SDO is to shape sports policy by putting local and national initiatives into practice and ensuring that all people of all ages and levels of ability have the opportunity to take part and develop their skills in sport.

There are different types of SDO, such as the generalist, sports partnership, local community, disability and sport-specific (Houlihan and White, 2002), who work for and with a range of stakeholders. The generalist SDO is one who develops a range of sports for a wide range of the population; the local community SDO serves the local community and develops local sports projects with and for local clubs and organizations; the sports partnership SDO serves a range of sports countywide and has links with GBoS; the disability SDO serves disability groups either from a local or national development perspective; the and sport-specific SDO serves a particular GBoS in developing and implementing strategies, making coach education courses available and servicing the needs of coaches and the GBoS as a whole.

Case study 2.2 – The role of the Sports Development Officer

Louise is a Regional Development Officer for a GBoS which is an Olympic sport and she is responsible for the development of this sport for the South of England. Louise undertook a Sports Development degree at the University of Wales Institute, Cardiff. At the time of undertaking this course in 1998, it was a new degree, which she thoroughly enjoyed. She knew this was a subject area that she wanted to pursue beyond the three years of the degree programme.

Having graduated, Louise avidly tried to pursue a sports development career, but many of the jobs that she was initially looking at and applying for were asking for a minimum of one year sports development experience. Louise initially took on several roles in the leisure industry hoping that eventually she would get a break into sports development. Her first role in sports development was as a Hockey Activator for the Active Sports programme in the Avon area for Sports South West. This was a great learning opportunity, as she had to initiate a programme of sports development activity where nothing had existed previously. Louise was provided with significant support from the GBoS (England Hockey), who provided a wealth of contacts locally which were pivotal to her development.

This role was only part-time but it had provided Louise with the necessary experience to move on and after two years she decided it was time to pursue a full-time sports development role working for a Local Authority. A two-year post was advertised working for Slough Borough Council as a generic Sports Development Officer and she was successfully recruited to the post. This post involved developing sport in the community for a range of sports, clubs and organizations, and also liaising with a range of stakeholders to implement local and national initiatives. Towards the end of this two-year period, and with no guarantees that the post would be extended, Louise decided to look around for new employment. A regional hockey development officer role was being advertised with England Hockey which Louise applied for, and after a rigorous interview and selection process she was appointed to the post in 2006. Within her current role as a Regional Development Officer for the England Hockey South Office, her remit is to oversee the coordination of the Level 1 and 2 hockey courses. This involves ensuring that appropriately trained coach educators and assessors are used, and that the courses are suitably located and accessible for potential coach candidates. On completion of the attendance aspects of the Level 2 Coach Award, candidates are required to complete a number of mentored hours post-course, and then apply to be assessed for their junior and adult coaching practical sessions.

When Louise first started the role she was tasked with identifying a number of county mentors of Level 2 or above to help support the Level 2 candidate coach through the qualification. Once the candidates had completed their assessments Louise was then responsible for arranging assessors to either go to the candidate's club to arrange an assessment, or organize a central assessment session, where it was ensured a number of assessors were available to assess the candidates.

On completion of the Level 2 Coach Award, Louise's role was to further support the coaches in making CPD opportunities accessible for progression to the Level 3 Coach Award (if deemed suitable by the assessors), and to other training opportunities to support the needs of the coach. A further role that Louise was tasked with was ensuring that all coach educators under the UKCC endorsement criteria undertook coach educator training in tutoring and assessing to ensure that England Hockey were standardizing processes and procedures to meet coaching requirements. This involved organizing modular training for coach educators to develop their tutoring, with a number being required to complete the Certificate in Tutoring Sport (CTS) and the Independent Assessment Practice in Sport (IAPS) portfolios.

Louise is also responsible for organizing a range of training opportunities for coaches in the South region including workshops and short courses. Louise is fulfilled in her role and enjoys supporting coaches and networking with a range of stakeholders in order to support the GBoS.

SUMMARY

The volunteer is an integral part of sport in the UK, and fulfils a range of roles including administrator, parent, official, helper, etc. A large part of the volunteer workforce in the UK is made up of sports coaches, who are a valued part of the sporting landscape in the UK. Volunteering can be viewed as a rewarding and valuable experience in the development of a coach, and many individuals start their coaching career as volunteers. The sports coach has a range of support networks available to them, and one of these networks is provided by a SDO, who either works for a GBoS, Local Authority or the local community. The SDO, along with their many other roles and responsibilities, provides opportunities for coaches to further their development in terms of providing access to coaching courses and CPD.

SEMINAR OR DISCUSSION QUESTIONS

1. What role does the volunteer sports coach play in supporting sport in the United Kingdom?
2. Highlight the roles and responsibilities of a Sports Development Officer.

KEY TERMS AND DEFINITIONS

- Coach educator – a senior coach who delivers coach education courses to candidate coaches.
- Continuing professional development (CPD) – attending further learning opportunities that support the coach and coaching practice.
- County Sports Partnership – provides a single system of delivery of sport in the community.
- Professional coach – one who is in paid full-time employment as a coach.
- Volunteer – an individual who helps others in sport through formal organizations such as clubs or governing bodies.

WEB LINKS

American Sport Education Programme (Volunteers) – www.ASEP.com
British Sports Trust – www.bst.org.uk
Clubmark – www.clubmark.org.uk
Institute for Volunteering Research – www.ivr.org.uk
Investing in Volunteers – www.investinginvolunteers.org.uk
Sport England County Sports Partnerships – www.sportengland.org/support_advice/county_sports_partnerships.aspx
Volunteering in Sport – www.volunteering.org.uk
Volunteer London 2012 – www.london2012.com/get-involved/volunteering/index.php

FURTHER READING

Bailey, S. (2007). *The Sports Source Book: A UK Directory of Sport.* Ch. 9: Volunteering in sport. Coachwise, SportsCoachUK, Leeds.
Cuskelly, G., Hoye, R. and Auld, C. (2006). *Working with Volunteers in Sport: Theory and Practice.* Routledge, London.
Houlihan, B. and White, A. (2002). *The Politics of Sports Development: Development of Sport or Development through Sport.* Routledge, London.

Chapter 3

Coaching and performance

CHAPTER OBJECTIVES

- Examine the impact that coaching has on performance.
- Explore what it is like coaching high performance athletes.
- Explore what is like coaching high performance athletes.
- Provide a case study of working in a high performance environment in basketball.
- Provide a case study of coaching high performance athletes in canoeing.

THE IMPACT COACHING HAS ON PERFORMANCE

Coaching has a significant impact upon sports performance, and is about improving performance at all levels (Crisfield *et al.*, 2003). A UK Sport survey during 2007 showed that "93% of athletes rated the coaching they had received was either very good or good and two thirds of the athletes surveyed wanted to stay with their current coach for the rest of their career, which was a desire more likely to be expressed by potential medal athletes" (SportsCoachUK, 2008n). This shows that coaching has a significant impact on sports performance at the elite level. However, it must also be remembered that these athletes started their careers at the grass roots level and therefore the impact of coaching throughout their career and at each stage of their development cannot be understated.

The coaching performance pathway for many coaches begins at the grass roots level, and if they are motivated and have the necessary skills, some progress to high performance coaching. Some athletes (ex-internationals) are fast tracked by their GBoS and have the opportunity to coach at the high performance level at the beginning of their coaching career because they have a wealth of experience and knowledge to impart. However, this is not always the case and it cannot be assumed that every ex-international athlete can make the transition to becoming a good coach.

Generally, at the grass roots level the coach will be introducing the athlete to the fundamentals of the sport, and at the high performance end of the spectrum the coach would be working a lot more intensively with the athlete, providing high levels of technical input and performance analysis, and developing and implementing individualized training programmes.

Lyle (2002) suggests that the conceptual framework of sports coaching concepts becomes much clearer if two distinct forms of coaching are recognized: sports participation and

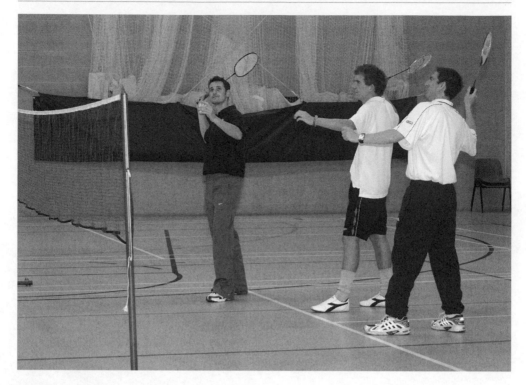

Photo 3.1 A coach instructing badminton players.

sports performance coaching. He further expands this contention by producing a model that shows a relationship between forms of coaching and boundary criteria (based on the fullest application of the coaching process) and which includes a progression of three forms of coaching. These forms of coaching include participation coaching, which is characterized by initiation into the sport and delivering basic skills, and accounts for the recreational and casual participant. Developmental coaching is characterized by rapid skills learning and engagement with a sport-specific competition programme. Thirdly, performance coaching is characterized by relatively intensive preparation and involvement in competition sport. A pictorial representation of this model is shown in Figure 3.1.

Figure 3.2 shows a suggested four-stage model that includes high performance coaching as another level. This should be viewed as a general model, and different sports may differ in terms of which level the coach works at, which may be through choice or lack of opportunities. The model can be best explained in terms of the coach moving from the foundation level of coaching through to high performance coaching, and each of these levels is matched by the progression of the performer. There is some flexibility in the model in terms of where the coach operates. For example, the club level performer could still be coached by a high performance coach. An example of this would be the coach who no longer has the desire to work at the top level and would rather develop young performers in the club environment. Another example would be the high performance coach working at club level, which maybe due to lack of opportunities at the higher level.

The nature of the sport may also dictate which level the coach is working at. If boxing is taken as an example, it could be that the club coach develops a boxer over a period of time

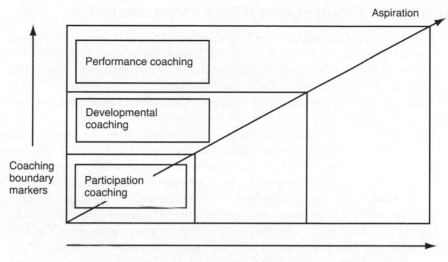

Figure 3.1 The relationship between forms of coaching and boundary criteria.
Source: Lyle (2002, Figure 3.5, p. 53).

at the amateur level. This could result in the boxer progressing through the ranks to win national titles, or alternatively turning professional. Being loyal, the boxer may want to keep the same coaching and management team that supported them through the early stages of their career, in which case the coach might find themselves working as a high performance coach in the high performance coaching environment, which is at ringside with their boxer, although they may still be classed as a club level coach.

Another consideration for this model is that some coaches may operate at all four levels at one time. This would possibly be the full-time professional coach who is working at national level, with a top club, carrying out some other club development coaching, and also delivering an after-school club coaching session.

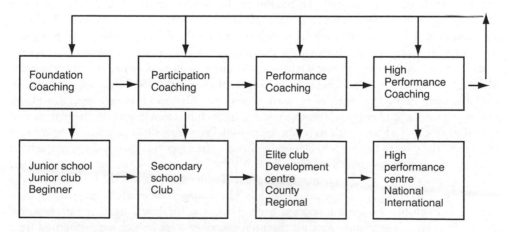

Figure 3.2 Four-stage coach-performer participatory model.

COACHING IN A HIGH PERFORMANCE ENVIRONMENT

High performance sport organizations exist in the United Kingdom to service and develop elite sport. These organizations are UK Sport, the English, Scottish and Welsh Institutes of Sport, the Sports Institute Northern Ireland and the British Olympic Association (see web links at the end of the chapter to access further information).

Many GBoS now operate with a High Performance Unit (HPU) whose sole focus is on their high performance athletes and high performance coaching staff. These HPUs not only utilize coaching expertise, they also draw on a range of disciplines to serve the high performance environment. This expertise will include specialists such as physiotherapists, physiologists, psychologists, doctors, strength and conditioning coaches and any other expertise that the HPU believes will have a positive impact on the development of the athlete and the coaching system that is being implemented. Goodbody (2008) suggests that one reason for England's 2003 rugby union World Cup victory was that Sir Clive Woodward gathered around him a team of experts, all of whom were able to contribute to the triumph of the team. The following case study highlights what it is like coaching in a high performance environment.

Case study 3.1 – Coaching in a high performance environment

Steve has played National League basketball and represented England at under-19 level. He coached a top National League team during the 1980s and 1990s and he has also coached a second division National League side. During this period he was involved in European competitions as well as domestic championships.

Steve is a Level 4 senior coach tutor and coach educator, qualified to deliver coaching qualifications up to Level 3. While coaching in the National League in all competitions he achieved a winning percentage of 62 per cent, which is highly rated. As an assistant coach during the 1980/1 season he won the National League 2 and the National Trophy, and in the 1981/2 season he won the National Cup. During the 1983/4 season, and still as assistant coach, he won National League 1, the National Cup and the Play-Off Championship. As head coach he won the National Cup during the 1982/3 season and in 1986 reached the National Cup final, also as head coach. Taking these achievements into account, Steve has extensive experience of coaching in the high performance environment. As an assistant and head coach, Steve spent nine years predominantly during the 1980s coaching professional and semi-professional basketball players, but at the same time he worked as a teacher of PE. Although the coaches in professional basketball were paid, it was however a high-risk coaching role that was very much sponsorship- and results-driven – hiring and firing was very common. Consequently, Steve made the decision early on not to become a professional coach, but to maintain a part-time status with the employment safety net of being a teacher. Although being in a high performance environment during the 1980s, the support systems available were limited in terms of utilization of sports science. However, specialist fitness equipment was utilized by Steve's management and coaching team to support the players, and a physiotherapist and osteopath were also employed. Private medical care was also provided for some of the players by the club. Generally though, the support team consisted of the head coach, assistant coach and the manager. Obviously the head and assistant coaches carried the coaching sessions, but the team manager had a much wider role and was the link between the coaching staff and the administration of the club. The manager was in a full-time paid position and was responsible for accommodation for the overseas (mainly American) professional basketball players, organizing work for the professional players (which supplemented their playing and sponsorship income), as well as guest appearances for the professional players, transport to and from venues, practice timings, work permits for the overseas players, being a direct link with the media wanting to talk to players and the coaches and working with TV companies for televised games. This is not an exhaustive list of responsibilities, but it does show that in a high performance environment there are a range of important roles and responsibilities.

Before coaching in the National League's top division Steve was playing and assisting with coaching at another National League side. The step up to coaching a top National League 1 side was a massive step for him in terms of the level of ability of players he was working with. This was the first time he had stepped into a professional sport environment, and he realized that this was a job where results mattered, and not just a recreational activity, and with this the pressure increased. Initially in this environment Steve found it difficult to establish a working relationship with the players, which was largely due to the player-coach credibility issue (the players possibly thought in terms of "What can an inexperienced coach tell us?" and questioned the level he had played or coached at). However, Steve indicated that coming in as an assistant coach to a US professional coach made the transition a lot smoother. Specifically, what he was able to contribute as the assistant coach ensured that the players understood where he was coming from in terms of a technical and tactical knowledge based perspective.

Steve found the psychological aspect of working in a high performance environment interesting, especially when dealing with the egocentric attitudes of the top players and their approach to the game. This he found frustrating and difficult to handle at times, especially on a day-to-day basis, but he also saw this as a "necessary evil". He understood that it was this trait that made them the players they were, and that you have to work with their egos rather than against them. A further role that Steve played was as a scout. An objective of this role was to glean technical and tactical information on opponents in preparation for the next match. These scouting reports were utilized to prepare the players to execute offensive and defensive plays and also used to inform practice schedules for the following week and beyond. The head and assistant coaches had specific roles in implementing these strategies, which left the players able to focus purely on execution rather than getting too involved in the analysis of the opposition.

In coaching at this level Steve also realized that the roles that each individual plays become more specific, and he found that he was dealing with experts in a wide range of roles. Steve considers that working in the high performance environment is thrilling because you are coaching players who can execute almost anything you ask of them. They are able to display a high level of technical skill, athleticism and decision-making ability. He also enjoyed the fact that game coaching became a game of chess, in that coaching strategies could be tested to the limit against other teams and coaches. Steve also considers that it was stimulating working with other high performance coaches and to have the opportunity to learn from them. He was able to see both ends of the coaching styles spectrum. He worked with a highly autocratic coach and a democratic coach, both of whom demonstrated considerable strengths in terms of their knowledge of the game.

Steve did acknowledge that there are some real challenges when coaching in a high performance environment. One of the main issues was losing because of not getting the preparation right, and travelling was also tiring. He could not make some of the European competitions because of other commitments, and it was this inability to be able to fully commit that he sometimes felt was a negative factor in working in the high performance environment. Moreover, there was a huge amount of time committed to coaching, which does impact upon family and social aspects of life.

Because of his positive experiences of coaching in the high performance environment, Steve would recommend and encourage young coaches to take on high performance coaching roles in order for them to gain experience. He feels that coaches should take the opportunities presented to them and that they should sometimes take risks in their coaching, because the coach may think "if only" later on down the line. However, young coaches should also be prepared for criticism, but this should be taken onboard as a learning process which will hopefully make the coach stronger, wiser and better the next time around. Steve is still involved in basketball as a coach educator, and he now combines his coaching skills with his role as a senior lecturer in HE.

Working with high performance athletes is rewarding but it also presents challenges for the coach in terms of commitment, time and travel. Many coaches in a range of sports aspire to work with high performance athletes and are happy dedicating their lives and career in the pursuit of performer and coach excellence, but it is not for everybody. An issue that might need to be considered in the UK is that when some high performance coaches retire, they retire at the top of their profession, when in fact their technical expertise and experience could be far better utilized at the junior level. If this experience and knowledge was delivered at the junior level then undoubtedly it would accelerate the learning of the aspiring junior performers. The next case study illustrates what it is like working with high performance athletes in canoeing and its respective disciplines.

Case study 3.2 – Coaching high performance athletes

Ian is a British Canoe Union registered coach, who has attained Level 5 coach status for Inland Water and Surf. He is also a Level 4 coach for Sea, and a Level 5 coach educator and assessor. In essence, he is at the highest level of coaching for his GBoS. Ian has 24 years coaching experience and has coached high performance athletes for the past 20 years. Early in his coaching career and as a teacher of PE, time off during the summer provided Ian with the opportunity to be more involved in coaching.

During the summer, high performance canoeists were offering to pay to be coached by Ian while he was working in the French Alps. For example, a canoeist would approach Ian with a specific environmental condition or coaching requirement. Ian would then deliver a coaching session appropriate to the needs of the performer dependent on their ability level and technical requirements. This may have entailed delivering a session in a grade 4 or 5 white-water river section (white-water river conditions are graded 1–6, with grade 6 the more difficult condition) or reinforcing or introducing a more advanced technique that the performer wanted to add to his or her repertoire. More of these types of opportunities were presented to Ian and his reputation soon grew, and it was during this early period of his coaching career that he began to aspire to work with high performance athletes, which he always viewed as the gold standard in terms of his coaching development.

Ian's professional philosophy in working with high performance athletes is to "keep it real", and to maintain currency and a detailed understanding of the sport. The perceived benefit that Ian gains from working with these athletes is that the athletes know what they want from the coach, which he finds very rewarding in terms of the performer coming to him for his expertise. Ian also highlights that the coach needs to know his business, because if you do not get it right the performer will know straight away. Ian also found that the meeting of specific needs of the athletes, working with the top end of the skill set and providing coaching solutions at a finer level were particularly rewarding and beneficial when working with high performance athletes. In terms of any highlighted problems when working in this environment, Ian thought that people management skills have to be highly developed, and he felt that peer pressure to display qualities and behaviours commensurate with the level and ability of a high performance coach was sometimes problematic. This can lead to high cognitive demands being placed on the coach, and the pressure of being held up as someone who knows what they are doing can sometimes be difficult. Ian also rated the physical requirements of working with high performance athletes, especially in his particular disciplines, as highly demanding. For example, continually being in the coaching environment in all sorts of weather, be it on the beach, river or lake can be tiring. Also, time and effort expended getting to venues can also be draining in terms of travelling to the venue, unpacking equipment, doing safety checks on equipment and assessing conditions, carrying out the coaching session, packing up equipment, debriefing and making the journey home. Many coaches can relate to this, but for this particular sport and in terms of the environment it is practised in, the demands on the coach can be seen as high. Ian does sometimes work with a team of coaches who are the same level as himself but have varying levels of experience, which he finds rewarding. However, unlike many team sports, this particular sport and its associated disciplines do not often have teams of coaches and in many cases the coach can be found operating in an individual capacity.

Although Ian is a highly qualified coach and coaches at the top level, he does also deliver sessions for different levels of ability, and like other coaches who coach at the grass roots level the coaching is pitched at a basic level. For the lower ability performer the environmental conditions are chosen very carefully and safety considerations are a major focus at this level. At the high performance level Ian mentions that the athletes are pushed harder and the practice strategies are much more rigorous. However, interpersonal and communication skills are not much different for the beginner or high performance athlete.

A focus for Ian in his coaching of high performance athletes is to strive for coach independence. Specifically this means that he does not want the performer to rely on the coach for instructions and to make decisions for them all of the time. This is also important bearing in mind the nature of the sport. The coach is not always going to be alongside the performer all of the time; they are often apart, and the environmental conditions, for example in canoe surfing, are constantly changing. Therefore, the performer has to be able to make decisions for themselves.

In terms of integrating sports science into his coaching, rudimentary psychological, physiological and biomechanical concepts are delivered, but in a way that are athlete-friendly and are not theoretically over-bearing. When working with high performance athletes Ian has to continually update himself on equipment design. For example, canoe shape, paddle blade design and safety equipment are constantly evolving and changing, which then requires the coach to understand that subtle changes in technical delivery have to be accounted for when coaching. This is coupled with a need to keep up to date with current underpinning knowledge of technical delivery and any changes that may be disseminated by international coaches after major competitions. Ian continues to work with high performance athletes and in coach education for his GBoS and still lectures at a HE institution.

SUMMARY

Coaching has a significant impact upon performance, and improves performance at all levels. High performance sport organizations exist in the UK to service and develop elite sport. These organizations are UK Sport, the English, Scottish and Welsh Institutes of Sport, the Sports Institute Northern Ireland and the British Olympic Association. Many GBoS now operate with a HPU, whose sole focus is on their high performance athletes, high performance coaching staff and delivery systems.

A coach can work at different levels from the foundation (grass roots) to the high performance coaching level. The coach can also work at different levels at the same time, which will depend on the sport they coaching and also on whether they are in a part-time or full-time coaching position. Coaches who have worked and who continue to work with high performance athletes in the high performance coaching environment find it very rewarding, but at the same time there are significant demands on their time. However, it is something that the coaches in the case studies have aspired to, and they recommend that any coach starting out in their career should also aspire to high performance coaching.

SEMINAR OR DISCUSSION QUESTIONS

1. Discuss the differences between foundation, participation, performance and high performance coaching, and how the level at which the coach operates may differ across sports.
2. Discuss the role of a High Performance Unit (HPU) in a GBoS of your choice.

KEY TERMS AND DEFINITIONS

- Developmental coaching – rapid skills learning and engagement with a sport-specific competition programme.
- Foundation coaching – coaching at the beginner or junior level.
- High performance coaching – coaching at the elite level.
- Individualized training plans or programmes – a specific training programme tailored to the needs of the individual performer.
- Participation coaching – initiation into the sport and delivering basic skills plus accounting for the recreational and casual participant.
- Performance analysis – analysing individual, team or squad performance utilizing a range of methods.
- Performance coaching – relatively intensive preparation and involvement in competition sport.

WEB LINKS

British Olympic Association – www.olympics.org.uk
British Association of Sport and Exercise Science – www.bases.org.uk
English Institute of Sport – www.eis2win.co.uk
UK Sport – www.uksport.gov.uk

FURTHER READING

Lyle, J. (2002). *Sports Coaching: A Framework for Coaches' Behaviour*. Routledge, London.
SportsCoachUK (2007b). Performance teams. *Coaching Edge*, 10(Winter), pp. 8–34.

Part 2

Effective sports coaching

INTRODUCTION

Part 2 of the book provides a broad outline of what constitutes effective sports coaching. Some concepts and processes that relate to effective sports coaching do not appear in this section – it was thought that they would better fit in chapters of their own for ease of comprehension. For example, being able to plan is part of being an effective sports coach, but it was felt that because of the importance of planning and the level of detail that should go into it, the subject warranted a section of its own.

Chapter 4 identifies and explains the skills, qualities, roles and responsibilities of the coach. Health and safety issues, risk assessments and the role of the coach are discussed at great length, together with two examples of how the coach should go through the process of accounting for health and safety before, during and after delivering a coaching session. Chapter 4 also outlines ethics and the code of conduct which the sports coach should abide by, and provides examples of codes of conduct for sports coaches in Canada, the UK and the USA. The chapter also looks at development of a coaching philosophy, which is supported by a case study of a practising elite level coach.

Chapter 5 is wide ranging and covers coaching behaviour and the impact it can have on the athlete and the coach; the differing coaching styles in which the coach can deliver; and understanding athletes' learning styles. Adaptation and differentiation will be explained with practical examples provided, along with what is effective communication and instruction: what is an effective demonstration; how to observe effectively; and how to how to provide feedback. These concepts will be considered from a broad theoretical point of view, and applied in the coaching context in order that the student can fully relate theory to practice.

Chapter 6 explains how practice is actually structured, in terms of how the coach delivers a coaching session, starting from the introduction (if the coach is working with a new group) to the reflect and review process at the end of the session. Chapter 6 also outlines practice principles – how the coach should run practices – and identifies the differing types of practice that are available to the coach, together with practical examples. At the end of each chapter suggested seminar or discussion questions and key terms and definitions are provided in order to support student learning. Web links and further reading are also provided in order for the student to carry out further research if required.

Chapter 4

The coach

CHAPTER OBJECTIVES

- Identification of the skills and qualities of a coach.
- Identification of the roles and responsibilities of a coach.
- Highlight health and safety issues and risk assessments.
- Ethics and the coach.
- Outline codes of conduct that exist for sports coaches in the UK, Canada and the USA.
- Explain a coaching philosophy.
- Provide a case study of a coach's coaching philosophy.

SKILLS AND QUALITIES OF A COACH

Throughout their career the coach will learn a range of skills and develop a range of qualities. Some of these skills and qualities may have already been developed through life and work experiences. For example, an individual who works in human resource management would be an excellent organizer, and a relationships counsellor would be a good communicator and listener. There are certain skills and qualities that underpin effective coaching and these are:

- ability to communicate effectively, which is inclusive of listening
- ability to provide impartial, timely and constructive feedback
- ability to be a good planner
- ability to be analytical
- ability to create and maintain a safe coaching environment
- possession of an enquiring mind in their coaching practice, and be motivated to increase their coaching skills and knowledge.

(Crisfield *et al.*, 2003).

These are generic skills and qualities and there are others which the coach may exhibit. One skill is having the ability to resolve disagreements, which may occur in the coaching environment. This is a particularly useful skill because unfortunately disputes do occur, for example between coaches and players, and players and officials, and the skill is in knowing when and how to diffuse the situation. A further skill that may also be required in this context is mediation. An example of where mediation might be needed is when the coach has to settle a dispute between his or her players over a specific role that they may have been given.

Developing as a role model is something that all coaches should strive for. Young sportspeople who aspire to be coaches when their playing career comes to an end need to be set a positive example in terms of how coaches conduct themselves, how they dress, and how they are seen to be fair, equitable and trustworthy.

The coach should also be knowledgeable of the technical and tactical requirements of their sport, and be able to provide effective and accurate demonstrations. They should also know that if they are unable to demonstrate, that a model (a technically able person in the group) can and should be used. This is a skill that should be developed over time, through practice, observing other coaches and by attending CPD workshops or events.

Transportation and getting young persons to and from venues can be an issue, especially if parents are unable to help, and a role that the coach may fulfil from time to time is that of a driver taking young athletes to and from training and competition. Understanding that being a "taxi driver" is sometimes part of the job is a quality, as is understanding that child protection issues also impact upon transportation issues, and therefore travel arrangements do have to be dealt with sensitively in terms of who is in a car with an adult.

A further skill that the coach needs to develop is the ability to observe, monitor and accurately assess performance in training and competition. This is required because accurate feedback is required in order for the performer to improve their performance, and providing and inviting feedback should form a major part of coaching practice. This will also facilitate development of an open, transparent relationship and keep communication channels open between the coach and performer.

The coach is required to conduct sessions in a safe environment, and they should be aware of all health and safety considerations. This skill should be honed very early on in the coach's career and the coach should also ensure that correct kit and equipment is worn and used, appropriate to the activity being conducted. The coach should ensure that young performers are provided opportunities to participate in appropriate levels of competition based on their age, ability and gender.

Arguably there are many more stresses and strains on young people in contemporary society than before, and young performers may have many areas of their life that are in competition with each other (family, education, sport, etc.). A further skill or quality that the coach may have to develop is the ability to advise young performers on achieving a balanced lifestyle (this will be looked at in more detail in Chapter 18). This may include advice on returning from injury and providing dietary advice, although ideally the coach should be referring the performer to a sports therapist and a nutritionist for this type of advice.

The coach should also be a good planner, as training plans (short-, medium- or long-term) must be delivered, and this is a fundamental skill that should be developed through experience over a period of time, and also by consulting with other coaches on how they plan. Arguably, there are many more skills and qualities that a coach is required to develop, and the ones that are highlighted here are certainly not an exhaustive list. The main message is for the coach to develop these skills and qualities over time. Some of these will not come easy, and will require some practice, but if the coach can get into good habits in the early stages of their career, it will facilitate their development.

ROLES AND RESPONSIBILITIES OF A COACH

The roles and responsibilities of a coach are as equally wide-ranging as the skills and qualities of a coach. The coach may find that they slip into one or more of these roles, depending on the coaching environment that they find themselves in, and with that comes the responsibility of the role.

The key responsibilities of a coach are:

- identifying and fulfilling the aspirations of the performer
- improving performance through a sequential, progressive, challenging and structured training and competition programme
- monitoring, reflecting upon and evaluating the efficacy of the programme in relation to the performer's aspirations
- creating a positive motivational environment both in training and competition
- creating a motivational environment that facilitates maintenance of involvement and maximizing potential in their chosen sport.

(Crisfield *et al.*, 2003)

In order to fulfil these responsibilities, there is a range of roles that the coach may have to undertake. Crisfield *et al.* (2003) identify roles in which the coach may undertake: an instructor who constructs and delivers practices; a motivator who creates a mastery-oriented motivational climate; a friend who supports the performer; a manager and administrator who looks after the day-to-day running of the squad or team and the administrative tasks; a social worker in providing pastoral support; a scientist in observation, analysis and seeking solutions to problems; a student in seeking out new learning opportunities to develop coaching knowledge and skills; and a protector ensuring that a coaching practice is carried out in a safe environment.

The coach may find that these roles are extended to include being a transport organizer in organizing transport for training, fixtures and tournaments; a disciplinarian in maintaining a fair, equitable environment and resolving conflict; a fitness trainer in developing fitness programmes appropriate to the needs of the individual; and a publicity agent in promoting and raising the profile of the club or organization that the coach is working for.

Again, these roles and responsibilities are not exhaustive, and will depend on the nature of the environment that the coach finds him or herself working in. For example, in an environment where the coach has limited access to support staff, they may find that they are wearing more than one hat at any one time. Conversely, if the coach is working in a high performance environment they will probably find that specific roles and responsibilities are delegated to other members of the support team, and the coach is only responsible for delivering activities and practices.

HEALTH AND SAFETY AND RISK ASSESSMENTS

Creating a safe environment is a crucial element in being an effective sports coach. The coach must be aware of health and safety at all times before, during and after coaching practice. It is essential for any coach to have attended a first aid course, which can be an Appointed Persons, Emergency First Aid or a St John Ambulance course. These courses provide the coach with the basic knowledge of how to respond to a range of emergency situations and how to treat common ailments or injuries. The coach should also ensure that they have

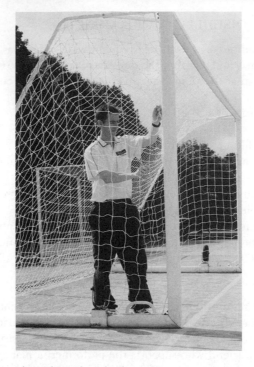

Photo 4.1 The coach going through a safety check.

adequate personal insurance cover at all times. Prior to delivering any coaching session the coach should make him or herself familiar with certain procedures, and also have access to a fully stocked first aid kit.

To illustrate health and safety issues when coaching, the following is an example of a netball coach using an indoor sports hall, and a rugby coach using an outdoor facility. A netball coach using the indoor sports hall for the first time should make themselves familiar with the normal operating procedures (NOPs) and emergency operating procedures (EOPs) for the facility before they start the session. The facility NOPs provide information on policies and procedures for minor incidents, which for example may be minor accidents that the facility staff may deal with on a daily basis. The facility EOPs provide information on policies and procedures for major incidents, such as fire and facility evacuation, which the coach should be conversant with because if any of these incidents occur knowledge of the location of exit and muster points is essential.

The netball coach should also conduct their own risk assessment prior to delivering the session. This may include assessing the risk to the coach or his or her participants from using equipment or from aspects of the use of the facility and rating the risk as high, medium or low. It is good practice to arrive at the venue early to ensure that all other equipment other than netball posts are cleared from the sports hall, the floor is clear of any fluid (which may be left from water bottles used by previous participants using the sports hall), there are no objects lying around that pose a risk to health and safety, and the equipment to be used is in good working condition. The coach should also make themselves familiar with the location of the nearest telephone, which in this example is probably at the reception.

On starting the session the coach should also ensure that personal health and safety is accounted for. For example, ensuring that the participants have the correct footwear and clothing, personal jewellery is removed and that any injuries or illnesses that anyone might have are accounted for. In the specific case of netball, fingernails should also be checked.

The coach should also outline the safety considerations for the activity, ensure that the space is used effectively in order that accidents do not occur, and conduct a full warm-up prior to starting the activity. On completion of the delivery of the session the coach should ensure a cool-down is conducted, all used equipment is packed away, and the facility is clear for whomever is going to use the sports hall next. If any injuries do occur then they should be reported to the reception staff where an accident report form should be completed and a copy made for the coach's own records.

It is essential that the coach has prior knowledge of any medical conditions that the participants may have (i.e. asthma, allergy to penicillin, etc.), which is of special importance when working with children, and in such cases the coach should also have the parents' contact details in the event of an emergency.

In the case of a rugby coach the process is similar, however, there are separate health and safety issues associated with an outdoor facility, and the nature of the sport also has to be considered. One of the main differences that affects the rugby coach in terms of health and safety is the pitch. The pitch should be checked for any dangerous objects, and if it is a night training session lighting should be adequate.

Weather conditions also have to be taken into consideration, in terms of the pitch potentially hardening with a night frost, and a range of inclement weather conditions that may affect the safety of the players. More often than not, access to a landline telephone is limited in this environment, but with the majority of people now using mobile telephones, this is not so much of a problem. It is also recommended that in this coaching environment the first aid kit is available at the side of pitch.

NOPs and EOPs will not be as extensive for a grass pitch facility, in comparison to an indoor facility. This is primarily because evacuation issues do not exist on a grass pitch (unless there is a fence surrounding the pitch) but it is still worth the coach checking if NOPs and EOPs exist for the facility that is being used. A risk assessment should still be carried out, and because of the physical demands that are placed on rugby players, an adequate warm-up appropriate to the nature of the activity is of special importance. If the rugby pitch does not have a facility with a reception, in the event of any accident it would be the responsibility of the coach to complete an accident report form and ensure that there is an access point for an ambulance if the need arises.

Health and safety issues and the coaching of children are important in terms of ensuring that they are wearing appropriate clothing, when the potential to get cold and wet is high during the winter.

Hopefully, this section has provided the student with an understanding of the health and safety issues that the coach has to be aware of when coaching. These checks may seem long and time consuming, but once the coach has gone through the correct process a few times, it becomes second nature. It is not worth cutting corners – the health and safety of the participants are of paramount importance when coaching.

This outline of accounting for health and safety issues is a useful guideline only and different facilities will require different approaches to health and safety. A suggested health and safety checklist, risk assessment and an accident report form are given in Appendices 1, 2 and 3 respectively. These are very basic forms, in which the criteria are very broad. However, as the coach develops his or her coaching expertise, and becomes more attuned to the importance of health and safety issues, these forms can be adapted to suit the coach's needs and the particular coaching environment that they find themselves in.

ETHICS AND THE COACH

The coach is faced with ethical and moral decisions on a regular basis. Within every relationship there is a power relationship (Zeigler, 1984) and the coach needs to consider who is exerting power in the coach-athlete relationship because there is the potential for coaches and athletes alike to abuse the relationship for monetary gain or recognition.

A coach of a female team might be faced with a moral dilemma if one of the players becomes pregnant and wants to carry on playing sport through the gestation period. The ethical issue involves questioning the right time during gestation to stop participating in sport, and who should make that decision, the coach or the player. What of the boxing coach, who knows that his or her boxer has the apolipoprotein E4 gene, which is a risk factor for chronic inflammation of the brain (Ophir *et al.*, 2005)? Should the coach with this knowledge let his or her boxer carry on boxing? Is it morally right for a male coach to have a sexual relationship with one of his female players or vice versa?

Ethics in sport can be defined as the "systematic application of moral rules, principles, values and norms [that] embrace the following core values of fairness, integrity, respect and equity" (Sport Scotland, 2003, p. 4). Each and every coach has a set of beliefs/morals which may centre on why they coach (a philosophy) or how they train their performers. Ethical behaviour actually takes moral strength, and it sometimes can take courage to resist pressures from short-term solutions, e.g. playing an injured player before the rehabilitation process is complete.

Another example is one of conformity: if unethical behaviour is endemic within a club or organization, does the coach conform to the status quo or stand up and abide by his or her own moral principles and speak out? Dulaney (2001) further suggests that the coach also a has moral obligation to maintain and preserve his or her integrity, to honour contracts, use professional expertise on an athlete's behalf and to maintain standards in the coaching profession.

CODES OF CONDUCT AND SPORTS COACHING

It is the coach's responsibility to abide by a code of conduct and behave in an ethical manner. Furthermore, coaches should have a good understanding of their legal obligations with regard to negligence, risk, duty of care, child abuse, insurance, transportation and drug use and abuse. Ignorance is no longer an acceptable excuse for any potential lapses of judgement, because information regarding these issues is widely available in the public domain (Crisfield *et al.*, 2003).

In different countries the Code of Conduct for Sports Coaches may vary in content, but the guiding principles are more or less the same. In Canada, the Canadian Association of Coaches has produced a Coaching Code of Ethics through their National Coaching Certification Program, which identifies four principles as "respect for participants, responsible coaching, integrity in relationships and honouring sport" (CAC, 2005). The United States Olympic Committee outline a Coaching Ethics Code which identifies six principles: "competence, integrity, professional responsibility, respect for participants and dignity, concern for others welfare, and responsible coaching" (USOC, 2008). For further information on Codes of Conduct for Sports Coaches in Canada and the USA, access the web links at the end of this chapter. Australia also has an extensive Code of Behaviour for Sports Coaches, and the relevant web link also appears at the end of this chapter.

In the UK many sports clubs, organizations and GBoS set out a code of conduct and an ethical framework which they expect coaches to adhere to. One of the first code of ethics was developed and published by the British Institute of Sports Coaches (BISC) (SportsCoachUK, 2001). The BISC code provided the value statement underpinning the National Vocational Standards (1992) for Coaching, Teaching and Instructing. The code is a framework and a series of guidelines rather than a set of hard-and-fast rules.

SportsCoachUK (2001) further developed this code into the Code of Conduct for Sports Coaches, which outlined the following four key principles: Rights, Relationships, Responsibilities (personal standards) and Responsibilities (professional standards).

- Rights: coaches must respect the rights of every individual to participate in sport regardless of age, ability, gender, race, creed, religious or sexual orientation.
- Relationships: coaches must foster positive relationships with athletes based on openness, honesty, trust, respect and equity.
- Responsibilities (personal standards): coaches must conduct themselves appropriately in the way they dress and act at all times.
- Responsibilities (professional standards): to maximize performance benefits for the athlete and create and maintain a safe coaching environment. Coaches must attain a high level of competence through qualifications and a commitment to continuous professional development that keeps them current with coaching practice.

(SportsCoachUK, 2001)

COACHING PHILOSOPHY

A coaching philosophy can be viewed as a set of moral beliefs that determine a coach's behaviour in a range of situations. Cross and Lyle (1999, p. 30) suggest that a coaching philosophy is a "comprehensive statement about the beliefs and behaviours that will characterize the coach's practice". Different coaches have different reasons (philosophies) for why they coach, which may be to win, to improve the performer or purely for their own enjoyment.

Some unscrupulous coaches have a philosophy of bending the rules, even to the extent of condoning the taking of performance enhancing drugs. For example, it has been well documented that during the 1970s and 1980s prior to the collapse of the Berlin Wall, Eastern European athletic and swimming coaches were routinely giving their athletes performance enhancing drugs without their knowledge and certainly without their full consent (Horizon, 2006).

A coaching philosophy can also exist within a team or a squad, and may be based around acceptable boundaries of what and what not to do in certain situations. A coach may also develop a team philosophy based around training principles, such as arriving at training on time, and around the team selection process and issues of training and over-training for young performers.

In essence, a coaching philosophy is what the coach believes in, based upon his or her own morals and beliefs. A coaching philosophy is determined by many factors, such as the beliefs the coach may already have, past experiences that may shape thought processes, influences from other coaches, family or friends, the knowledge the coach has and the situation that they find themselves in. Moreover, the emotions that were felt in a previous experience, and any emotions felt in a present experience may also affect any decision that is made by the coach. A suggested coaching philosophy affective model is shown in Figure 4.1.

Case study 4.1 – Development of a coaching philosophy

Sue is an England Hockey Level 3 coach, a FIH Junior Master Coach and a coach educator, tutor, assessor and mentor. Sue has been coaching for 37 years, and has coached at national, regional and National League levels. Sue started coaching at the age of 16 and in order to be coached herself she was required to help coach juniors at her local club, which was the main reason she started coaching at such an early age. The reason why Sue coaches is for the love of her sport; she enjoys imparting knowledge and understanding of the game, and the interaction with young players. She also enjoys creating a positive learning environment and developing a two-way communication process with players.

Sue is dedicated to the process of coaching, and really enjoys engaging in all aspects of this, especially the reflect and review process. A further reason why she coaches is that it gives her structure in her life, knowing that she has to go out and coach certain evenings and that her weekends are also accounted for, which she also sees as being institutionalized in a positive way.

Sue highlights player development as the single most important focus in her coaching. This she feels helps the player become more focused as an individual on how they acquire skill and apply knowledge and understanding. Sue feels it is important to get players to understand the "when and why" along with the "how" to execute skill, which she believes empowers the player in their own decision making.

Although player development is important, Sue also likes winning; she feels that there is no point in turning up if you do not want to win a game. However, she feels that you do learn more about yourself as a coach and about your players when you lose games. We can all feel positive and happy when winning, but it is how you deal with losing that gives you a greater insight into yourself and your players.

Sue also coaches for her own self-development and believes in looking outside of her own

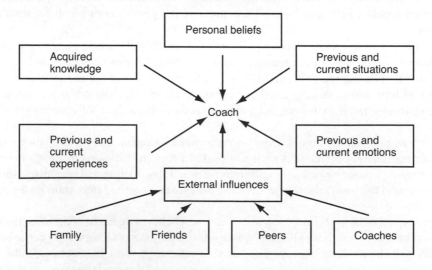

Figure 4.1 Coach philosophy affective model.

sport and observing coaching practices in other sports. This enables her to see if skills and strategies used in these other sports would be useful to implement in her own sport.

Sue enjoys her coaching, but it sometimes can be a chore, especially when different agendas are displayed by players, for example when they come to a training session with preconceived ideas about how they should be coached and at what level they should be coached at. There have been some players whose ego has exceeded their ability, so their perception of what they can achieve is incorrect. Sue describes this in another way: some players have played at a high level almost through default, and they are not sure how they got to that level. Sue feels that no real form of learning had taken place for the player; it was almost as if they had become unconsciously competent in their sport.

Sue believes in fair play, and feels that it is crucial the coach is supportive of those officiating, and that players should understand officials' roles more. There is no such thing as a perfect player and officials are not perfect either, and players should understand this. Sue's philosophy means she will substitute players who do not adhere to the rules and accept officials' decisions. She believes that fair play and sportsmanship need to be taught to young people earlier in their sporting careers; social etiquette should also be developed as it was many years ago, and young people should make an attempt to officiate more.

In terms of athletes over-training, Sue's believes the player comes first at all times and feels that there has to be a player pathway framework. She is concerned that some coaches are more interested in their own success, and that they do not consider the individual, meaning that over-training, over-playing, injury and consequently burnout do occur. Sue feels that there should be a balance between training, playing and other areas of a player's life. Coaches should take on a more holistic view and look at all aspects of player development, which is something you are only going to get from player-centred coaches, not from ego-centred coaches. Sue continues to coach, and is still involved in coach education delivering Coach Award courses, assessing and mentoring coaches.

SUMMARY

The skills and qualities of a coach are multi-faceted, and these need to be developed over time. The coach may also find that they have a multitude of roles and responsibilities to fulfil, especially if they are working in isolation, but these roles and responsibilities are more likely to be shared if they are working in a high performance environment. Creating a safe environment is crucial to being an effective sports coach, and the coach is required to have extensive knowledge of health and safety issues.

It is the coach's responsibility to check the facility he or she is working at, account for player personal safety, and carry out regular risk assessments, as well as to have insurance and a first aid qualification. It is the responsibility of the coach to conduct him or herself in an ethical manner, and to abide by a Code of Conduct for Sports Coaches. Lapses of moral judgement are no longer an excuse, as plenty of information exists in the public domain that can inform the sports coach on a range of ethical and code-related issues. All GBoS have a code of conduct by which they expect their coaches to abide by, and SportsCoachUK also promotes a Code of Conduct for Sports Coaches.

Most coaches will have a coaching philosophy, which is based around their belief system. Coaches will have different philosophies, depending on where they place the emphasis in their coaching, which could be on a desire to win, self-development, player development or on ensuring that the players enjoy themselves.

SEMINAR OR DISCUSSION QUESTIONS

1. Identify and explain the differences between the skills and qualities and the roles and responsibilities of the coach.
2. Discuss the issues surrounding a coaching philosophy.

KEY TERMS AND DEFINITIONS

■ Balanced lifestyle – having a lifestyle that is more or less equal in all parts and includes sport, family, friends, finances, education, etc.
■ Coaching philosophy – a moral set of beliefs that determine a coach's behaviour in a range of situations.
■ Code of conduct – a set of values and principles that guide coaching practice.
■ Emergency operating procedures (EOPs) – a policy which provides information on fire, evacuation and emergency procedures.
■ Mediator – someone who intervenes to settle a dispute.
■ Normal operating procedures (NOPs) – a policy which provides information on the day-to-day running of a facility.
■ Risk assessment – a system which identifies items and situations that may cause accidental injuries or health problems.
■ Training plan – an organized schedule of coaching over a period of time.

WEB LINKS

Australian Sports Commission (Coaches' Code of Behaviour) – www.ausport.gov.au/participating/coaches/education/ethics/coachbehaviour
Canadian Association of Coaches (Code of Conduct) – www.coach.ca/eng/ethics
United States Olympic Association (Coaching Ethics Code) – www.asiaing.com/united-states-olympic-committee-coaching-ethics-code.html

FURTHER READING

Crisfield, P., Cabral, P. and Carpenter, F. (2003). *The Successful Coach; Guidelines for Coaching Practice* (3rd edn). SportsCoachUK, Leeds.
Cross, N. and Lyle, J. (2002). *The Coaching Process: Principles and Practice for Sport*. Butterworth-Heineman, Oxford
McNamee, M. J. and Parry, S. J. (1998). *Ethics and Sport*. Routledge, London.

Chapter 5

Analysing coaching concepts

CHAPTER OBJECTIVES

- Define and explain coaching behaviour.
- Identify and describe leadership styles.
- Identify and describe different coaching styles.
- Identify and describe different learning styles.
- Describe the concepts of adaptation and differentiation.
- Explain communication and instruction.
- Explain what an effective demonstration is.
- Explain how the coach should observe effectively.
- Explain feedback.

COACHING BEHAVIOUR

Coaching behaviour can be defined as the behavioural responses exhibited by the coach in response to his or her performer's behaviour (Smith *et al.*, 1977). The way the coach behaves and interacts in any given situation with his or her performers is an interesting concept, and many coaches are unaware of the effect their behaviour can have on the behaviour of their performers.

Coach behaviour can be influenced by the coach's perception of the performer, and vice versa. Some coaches can gravitate towards certain performers for a number of reasons, such as the coach perceiving the performer to be skilful or a highly confident individual. The reverse of this is the coach who ignores the performer they perceive to be less skilful or lacking in confidence. This behaviour may have a negative impact on the performer, making them less confident because the coach is taking no notice of them, and consequently become an issue in the performer-coach relationship.

Furthermore, the coach needs to be aware of the effects of presenting non-verbal communication to the performer. For example, body language and facial expressions (non-verbal communication) can give a lot of information away as to the coach's feelings, and performers will pick up on these non-verbal signals.

The observing and recording of coach behaviour has grown into a science, and one of the most widely used measuring systems is the Coach Behaviour Assessment System (CBAS) which was developed to allow direct observation and coding of coaches' actions (Smith *et al.*,

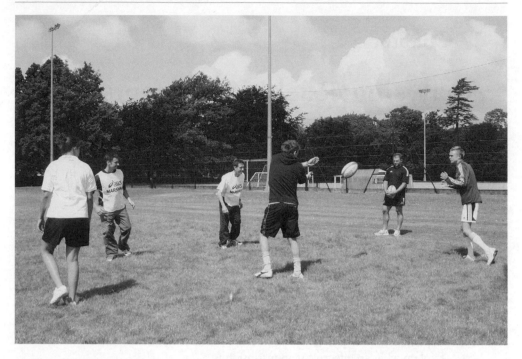

Photo 5.1 The coach exhibiting negative body language and behaviour.

1978). The CBAS is comprised of 12 behavioural categories, which are over-arched by the two major constructs of reactive behaviours and spontaneous behaviours.

Reactive behaviours are responses to athlete or team behaviours (Smith *et al.*, 1977) which are divided into the sub-constructs of desirable performance, reactions to errors and response to misbehaviours, and have associated responses that the coach will exhibit. The responses associated with desirable performance are positive reinforcement and non-reinforcement. The responses associated with reactions to errors are error dependent motivation, error dependent technical instruction, punishment, punitive or ignoring errors, while the response associated with misbehaviours is keeping group control (Smith *et al.*, 1977).

An example of the coach reacting to a desirable performance by a basketball player might be providing positive reinforcement or reward, such as "Well done, that was a good lay up", or non-reinforcement, in which the coach does not react to points being scored. In the sub-construct reaction to errors, an example of error dependent motivation would be the coach saying "Keep your head up and keep going" after an error by a player. Regarding error dependent technical instruction, the coach might provide technical feedback to the player after he or she has made an error. For example, a volleyball player may have made an error on the dig, and the coach's reaction might be "Bend your knees more and keep your eyes on the ball".

Regarding punishment, this is a negative reaction by the coach following an error and could be either a verbal or non-verbal response. A verbal response could be the coach berating the performer, and a non-verbal response could be a negative facial expression, a folding of arms or a turning away. Punitive and punishment coach behaviours can occur together, and this may include the coach telling an athlete repeatedly to get the skill right. For example, "How many times have I told you to mark that player?".

In the final sub-construct, the response to misbehaviours, the coach's reaction should be to keep control. An example would be a soccer coach with a large group of children in a training session and who needs to maintain control of the group for health and safety reasons. There could be some children at the back of the group being less than attentive when the coach is trying to give group feedback and there will be a need for them to re-focus their attention.

Spontaneous behaviour is initiated by the coach and is not in response to the player's behaviour (Smith *et al.*, 1977). It can be divided into two sub-constructs: performance relevant and performance irrelevant responses. Both of these have a specific behaviour associated with them. Performance relevant behaviour consists of general technical instruction, general motivation and organization, and performance irrelevant behaviour consists of general verbal and non-verbal communication.

An example of performance relevant general technical instruction is informing a cricket player how to bat or field, a bowler which bowling technique to use or setting up the fielders to account for either a left or right handed batsman. In terms of general motivation, unlike error dependent motivation, this is not a response to specific actions by the players (Smith *et al.*, 1977). This type of behaviour is more democratic in its response, being more of a request than an explicit instruction. For example, the coach may say "Keep going lads, let's try and get a few more runs and a couple more wickets". In terms of performance relevant organization, the coach behaves in an organizational manner. For example, reading out team lists prior to the start of a game, changing tactics or organizing the order of penalty takers in a penalty shoot-out in soccer.

The second spontaneous behaviour sub-construct is performance irrelevant behaviour and consists of general verbal and non-verbal communication, which in its simplest form is the general interaction of the team or group and has nothing to do with training, competition or performance. This type of behaviour will include "banter" and communication regarding social issues (family, friends, social activities, etc.) outside of the sporting environment.

LEADERSHIP AND THE COACH

Leadership is another interesting concept that requires some attention and has implications for effective sports coaching. It could be argued that a coach needs to be an effective leader in order to fulfil the group objectives, or to guide the individual performer towards his or her ultimate goal. But what makes an effective leader? In cricket, England Captain Michael Vaughan inspired his team to an Ashes victory in 2005 and in the following competition Ricky Ponting, the Australia Captain, inspired his team to win back the Ashes from England. What qualities did these leaders have?

During the 2008 Beijing Olympics the British cycling team had unprecedented success, winning eight gold, four silver and two bronze medals. What leadership qualities did their coaching staff possess that inspired the cyclists to this stunning medal haul? In 2009 Brian O'Driscoll inspired Ireland to their first Grand Slam for 61 years. What leadership qualities did he possess? Were these leadership qualities any different to those of Michael Vaughan and Ricky Ponting?

Nick Nurse, who was the highly successful Head Coach and General Manager of the Brighton Bears basketball team in the UK developed a leadership style that involved all his players in the early stages of the decision-making process, providing them with some sense of ownership, and promoted a culture of personal growth and having the ability to adapt (Nurse, 2003). Were these qualities of an effective leader? Could it have also been due to the willingness of the group to accept a culture that promoted ownership?

Different theories have been proposed to provide a framework with which to understand effective leadership. One of these theories is known as trait theory and has its origins in the "great man" theory of leadership, which suggests that certain leaders have personality traits and characteristics that make them ideally suited for leadership (Case, 1998). Another theory is the theory of universal behaviours, which holds that successful leaders have certain universal behaviours, and once these behaviours are identified, they can be taught to potential leaders everywhere (Cox, 2007). Another group of theories are known as situation-specific or contingency theories, and these suggest an interaction between the leader and the situation (Cox, 2007).

Chelladurai (1980) extended the notion of leadership in coaching, and developed the Multi-Dimensional Model of Leadership. Chelladurai's model identifies satisfaction and performance as two outcomes of leadership and holds that the behaviours that determine these outcomes are either prescribed, preferred or actual leader behaviour (Horn, 2008). Prescribed leader behaviours are coaching behaviours that are aligned to the accepted philosophy of the team or athletes. For example, the coach would be expected to behave in a certain professional manner when coaching children and those behaviours are formed by the philosophy and/or code of conduct of the organization or coaching environment in which the coach is working.

Preferred leader behaviours are behaviours preferred by the athletes. For example, it might be expected that the coach is part of the social circle that meets up after training and competition, or that the coach, in accounting for all individual needs, is expected to utilize a range of coaching styles in training and competition. Actual leader behaviours are those behaviours that the leader exhibits irrespective of the expectations and philosophy of the athletes or team. In terms of the actual qualities that great leaders possess, there is no exact or definitive set of qualities, but this has not stopped a whole host of theorists, authors and academics adopting theoretical approaches that try to isolate them.

This author suggests that the qualities of an effective leader summarized by the Synergy Institute (Loo, 2009) is a good place to start. They will be: a lateral and forward thinker; passionate and compassionate; true to their own values; a risk-taker; action orientated; a builder of outstanding teams; a role model; a learner; an effective communicator and listener; highly competent; intuitive; a mentor, gracious in victory and defeat.

COACHING STYLES

A coaching style is the way in which the coach delivers his or her coaching session and in part is dependent on their philosophy of coaching. A coaching style will vary from person to person and situation to situation as the coach adapts their behaviour to meet the specific needs of the performers. Quite often coaching styles are placed on what is known as a continuum, from the autocratic command style where the coach makes all the decisions for the players, to the more democratic interactive style where the players discuss and negotiate issues (Lyle, 1999; Martens, 1987), through to the laissez-faire style, which provides little or no instruction or guidance and leaves the performer to get on with the sport.

There are advantages and disadvantages of these styles. Different styles are appropriate to different situations and individuals, and suit different learning styles (learning styles are discussed in the next section), although it is certainly not ideal to use the laissez-faire style. An example of a coaching styles continuum is shown in Figure 5.1.

There are times when the coach will need to be autocratic in organizing a large group of children or when they are in unsafe situations; equally there will also be times when the coach

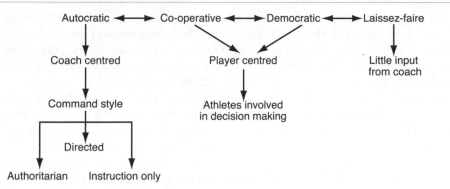

Figure 5.1 Coaching styles continuum.

wishes to stand back and observe performance and develop a more questioning approach, which is more democratic in nature. Effective coaching occurs when the coach is able to vary his or her style, recognizing when each style is required for any given situation.

Operating between each end of the continuum is sometimes referred to as the cooperative style, which offers leadership while encouraging performers to engage in the decision-making process (Martens, 1987). This delivery style also allows the athlete to take more responsibility for their own learning, which in essence is an athlete-centred approach. Many coaches feel comfortable delivering autocratically because it allows them to be in charge of the session (Crisfield *et al.*, 2003) but this does not lend itself to an inclusive, coach-athlete joint decision-making approach. However, as the coach becomes more experienced, confident and knowledgeable they will begin to understand that different styles are required depending on the coaching environment they are in (Crisfield *et al.*, 2003).

LEARNING STYLES

A learning style can be defined as "the complex manner in which, and conditions under which, learners most efficiently and most effectively perceive, process, store and recall what they are attempting to learn" (James and Gardner, 1995, p. 20). In the context of sport, it is the coach's responsibility to maximize individual athletes' performance by considering a range of factors (Owens and Stewart, 2004), and understanding and accounting for athletes' needs in terms of learning styles is essential for effective learning to take place. If the coach only accounts for one style or only delivers in his or her own preferred style, then the potential for ineffective learning to take place is likely.

Dunn *et al.* (1987) have identified five major variables that affect learning styles that the coach might consider when delivering his or her coaching session: the environment, societal factors, physiological and psychological factors and brain functioning. The practice environment changes constantly in terms of light, noise and temperature. If the weather is cold and wet the coach may not be able to use a coach board showing diagrams of the practice, which might not suit the activists (see below) in the group.

The performer may also be constrained by physical capability (fitness levels), which impacts not only upon their learning style but also on their ability to actually execute a skill. Parents, coaches and peers also influence the way an athlete thinks and learns, which can be considered a societal variable, and the psychological variables that might impact upon an athlete's learning style include motivation, concentration and confidence levels.

Brain functioning is an interesting aspect when accounting for athletes' learning styles because of the suggested mismatch in hemispheric brain functioning between the coach and athlete. Cowan (2005) suggests, in terms of left and right brain theory, athletes are right brain dominant, and display the characteristics of being creative, reactive and non-analytical. Coaches however, are suggested to be left brain dominant, and display the characteristics of being logical, analytical and critical. Cowan (2005) goes on to suggest that because of this mismatch in thinking, communication may become an issue, as right brained athletes prefer visual and kinaesthetic communication to the verbal criticism coaches often give them.

Many theorists have proposed models to explain the different learning styles that exist in an individual. However, the most notable among them are Peter Honey and Alan Mumford, who have developed a four factor framework, which lends itself to be applied to the coach-athlete relationship and coaching practice in a manner easy to understand. The four factors that make up Honey and Mumford's framework are Activist, Pragmatist, Reflector and Theorist. In order to accommodate the visual learning student, Figure 5.2 shows the interaction between the coach and athlete in terms of Honey and Mumford's four learning styles, signifying that the coach is responsible for accounting for all four learning styles.

Rather than explain the four different learning styles in written form, four separate diagrams have been constructed to provide a visual representation of their characteristics which have been adapted from Honey and Mumford's theories and characteristics of learning styles. Figure 5.3 shows the Activist's characteristics, Figure 5.4 shows the Pragmatist's characteristics, Figure 5.5 shows the Reflector's characteristics and Figure 5.6 shows the Theorist's characteristics.

So what does this mean for the coach and how can the coach structure their delivery and organize practices to account for the four different learning styles? Driscoll (2005) suggests the coach should focus on the performer as well as performance and should vary their language and approach to match the different learning styles of the performer.

There are certain strategies that the coach can use to account for each individual style in order to deliver the session effectively. Figure 5.7 shows the relationship between learning styles and the strategies that coaches can use to account for the performer's individual needs. To ensure that the coach maximizes the team or individual's potential, coaches need to understand these styles and integrate them when delivering in the practice and competitive environment (Owens and Stewart, 2004).

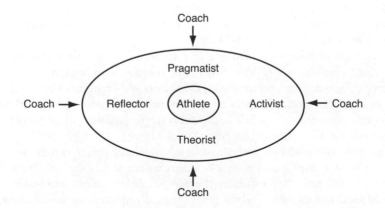

Figure 5.2 Coach-athlete learning styles interaction.

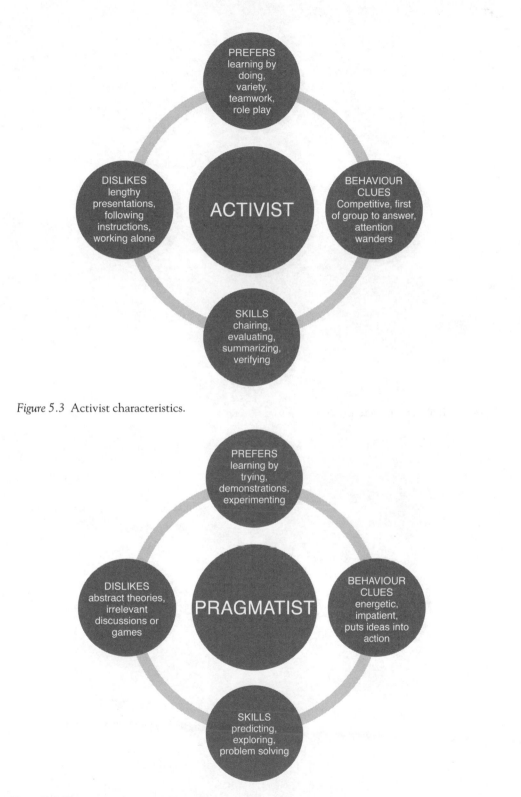

Figure 5.3 Activist characteristics.

Figure 5.4 Pragmatist characteristics.

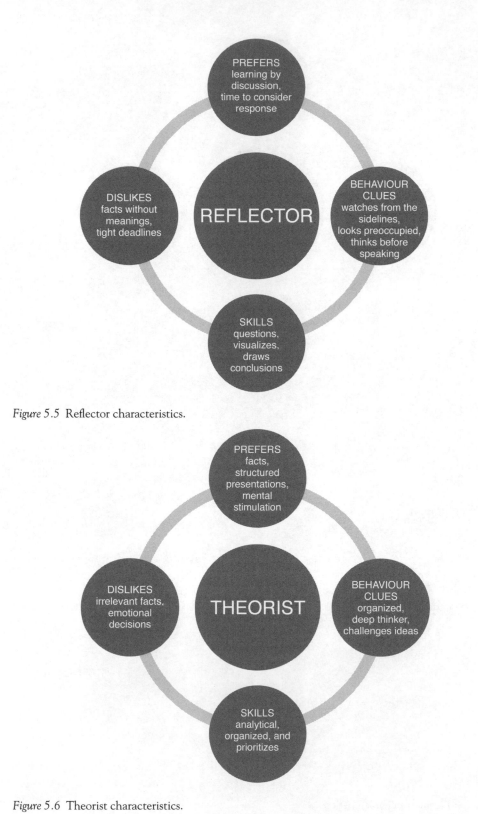

Figure 5.5 Reflector characteristics.

Figure 5.6 Theorist characteristics.

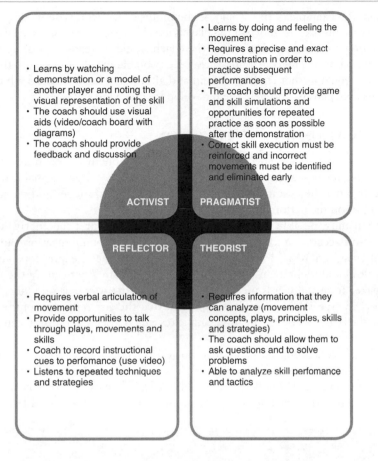

Figure 5.7 Learning styles and coaching strategies model.

ADAPTATION AND DIFFERENTIATION

The coach will at times need to adapt the coaching environment to meet the needs of his or her performers. This will depend on a number of factors, which include group size, group composition, ability, fitness, skill level and the coach's experience.

The STEPS concept (England Hockey, 2006) – Space, Task, Equipment, Position and Speed – is a good mnemonic to remember for how the environment can be adapted to account for a range of needs. Space relates to adapting the size of the practice area; Task relates to adapting the complexity of the activity; Equipment relates to adapting equipment; Position relates to adapting the position or number of players in the practice; and Speed relates to adapting the intensity of the activity to suit the needs of the athlete. The coach will also find they have to adapt their coaching and communication style when working with different groups (Crisfield *et al.*, 2003). Specifically, working with disabled groups will require a totally different coaching and communication style to working with able-bodied groups, and almost certainly adaptation will have to be considered.

A further consideration when adapting the coaching environment is the concept of differentiation. In basic terms differentiation is the coach altering the pace, space or the degree of complexity of the skill for those performers who are more or less able than others in the group. An example of this would be the tennis coach who is delivering a session on serving to six tennis players. If two of the players are able to execute the serve efficiently, and the other four are having problems, then the coach would increase the task complexity for the more able players. The coach may direct the two able players to execute the serve and volley, which would further challenge them and allow the coach to spend a bit more time with the less able players, and help them develop their serving skill.

COMMUNICATION AND INSTRUCTION

Being able to communicate effectively is a crucial component of coaching practice. The coach might be the most astute technician and tactician, but if they are unable to effectively communicate what they want their performers to do, the techniques and tactics would be completely lost on the performers.

The coach must be able to present information clearly and succinctly, and provide appropriate and accurate information (Robinson, 2006b). Communication can be divided into verbal (instruction) and non-verbal (body language, facial expressions and gestures) (Martens,1987) and Mehrabian (1968) suggests that we gain 7 per cent of the information from a speaker from the words used, 38 per cent from the way it is said, and 55 per cent from the way the speaker behaves. It is important that the coach is aware of the non-verbal information he or she is communicating, and takes care that it is not misinterpreted by their players.

How a coach communicates can affect motivation, confidence, concentration, anxiety levels, the athlete's feelings and behaviours, skill acquisition and the coach's ability to provide feedback on performance (Weinberg and Gould, 2007). When using verbal messages, Martens (2004) suggests that the coach must avoid making assumptions that the athlete understands

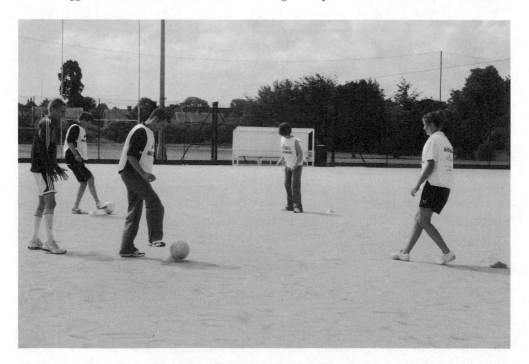

Photo 5.2 A coach instructing a group of soccer players.

what is being said or asked of them, give time for the athlete to interpret the coaching points or tactical information and repeat verbal cues if required in order to clarify or reinforce coaching points. The coach should also consider the tone of voice he or she uses when communicating. If the coach were to deliver in a monotone voice all the time the performer may well switch off – the coach should be enthusiastic.

Physical messages such as facial expressions, hand gestures and body movements, posture, body contact, spatial distance, clothes and appearance will also be interpreted in a positive or negative way by the performer. If the coach turns up in sandals, chinos, a baseball cap, unkempt and unshaven then the performer will instantly form an opinion, especially if they have not met the coach before, and in this particularly case it could be argued that the performer would not form a particularly good opinion of the coach. Being an effective communicator not only relies on the coach providing information, it also entails the coach being an effective listener (Martens, 2004). To be an effective listener Raygor and Wark (1970) propose that the following mnemonic can be used:

L – Look interested in what the speaker is saying.
I – Involve yourself in the communication process by questioning what you do not understand or what you want clarified.
S – Stay on target and try not to let the conversation drift off on a tangent.
T – Test your understanding – what does this information mean to me?
E – Evaluate the message – what are the good and not so good points?
N– Neutralize your emotions and try not to make judgements.
S – Self-reflect – could I on reflection have responded better?

There are certain strategies available to the coach to optimize communication, which include changing the group or team composition, restructuring and re-allocating group tasks and managing players' communicative behaviour (Hanin, 1992). Another strategy for optimizing communication between the athletes and the coach is the use of team-building exercises. These can include setting up exercises that optimize group work in the pre-season phase of training or going away on an organized team-building weekend in which the team participates in a range of tasks designed to foster group cohesion.

Hanin (1992) further suggests that for optimizing communication in training the coach should organize practice sessions that are physically and mentally stimulating and are focused on group success. Hanin adds that the coach should also ensure that practice sessions are goal-oriented, tension free and provide the athletes with the necessary skills to cope with training and competitive stress.

DEMONSTRATIONS

Having the ability to demonstrate is crucial in coaching practice, and the coach is required to have a good understanding of the technical aspects of their sport in order to demonstrate effectively. If, however, the coach is unable to demonstrate themselves, they should use a model (a skilled player) who is capable of performing the task, or use a video recording of the skill being performed so that the individual or group can reproduce the skill effectively. Confucius is said to have said "a picture paints a thousand words", but a closer translation of the original Chinese is "one showing is better than one hundred sayings". There is no more accurate a statement than this when it comes to coaching practice. If a demonstration is not provided and the skill is only verbalized then the potential for error in terms of reproducing the skill exists. Communicating the technical requirements of the skill is not enough, as it can lead to misinterpretation and does not accommodate the visual learner.

A demonstration provides appropriate information for developing a memory template which is technically correct. It also provides precise information of what can and cannot be done within the limitations of the body and equipment being used and, finally, a demonstration provides information about how movement is to be coordinated.

Bandura's (1977) Observational Learning Theory provides an explanation of how we learn by observing demonstrations, and suggests four sub-processes are critical: salience, memory and skill reproduction, desire and motor capability. Specifically, the performer should attend to the relevant (salient) technical information and the coach must reinforce the coaching points in order that the performer can perform and commit the skill to memory (memory and skill reproduction). The coach also has to consider whether the performer is motivated (desire) and whether they have the physical attributes (motor capability) to perform the skill.

Although the coach should demonstrate at key times during the session to reinforce coaching points, a demonstration should be provided at the start of the session, in order to give the general idea. Christina and Corcos (1988) suggest there are at least three times when a coach should demonstrate a skill: prior to the athletes performing the skill; at key points throughout the practice; and at the end to reinforce skill development. If the skill is complex, the coach should start off with the basic movement then add further elements of the skill bit by bit until the whole skill is able to be practised.

Hardy and Mawer (1999) propose that an effective demonstration is determined by certain characteristics:

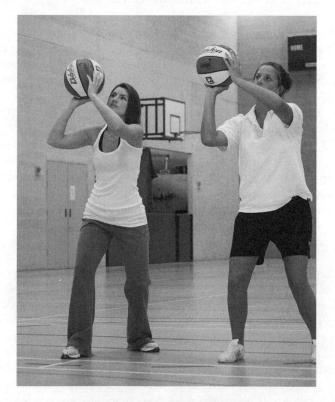

Photo 5.3 The coach on the right demonstrating a basketball skill.

1. Verbal information must be provided to support the demonstration.
2. The practice should be set up beforehand.
3. The movement or practice should be put into the context of the performance or game.
4. The demonstration should be accurate.
5. The demonstration should be organized in order for:

- The performer can see, hear and understand.
- Plenty of practice opportunities are made available.
- The coach is able to observe, monitor, feedback and correct errors.
- Performers practise the task as demonstrated.

When verbal information forms an element of the demonstration the coach must be careful not to overload the performer with too much information. The coach has to consider that the performer is taking in visual information as well as verbal information, therefore it is suggested that instruction be kept to a minimum. However, Schmidt (1991) suggests that instruction is an essential element of learning that provides useful and important information and can be used to emphasize correction of errors in performance.

The verbal information that is presented to the performer should be pitched at the ability of the performer (do not use jargon with young performers) and should be technically correct and relevant to the skill being demonstrated. Although instruction is time-saving, at the same time it can be often overused, and coaches can find themselves talking for far too long about the technical requirements of the skill when in an ideal world the performers should be practising the skill.

A question that arises when providing demonstrations is whether the skill should be demonstrated in slow motion or at the correct speed at which it is executed. There are some sports (boxing combination punching, some gymnastic routines, etc.) that are performed too quickly for the performer to perceive and reproduce the skills effectively and accurately. A strategy that the coach might employ is to demonstrate the skill in slow motion at first, but the performer must as soon as possible practise the skill at the correct speed of execution.

OBSERVATION

In its simplest form observation is concerned with what to look for in a logical order and the coach needs to consider whether the problem that he or she is observing is either technical or tactical, depending on the sport (Robertson, 2002). The more experienced coach sees that skill execution is correct and leaves it alone, is able to see ineffective technique, recognizes why it is occurring and knows how to correct technical errors. Observation is a key skill for the coach to develop. This particular skill (some coaches may view this as an art) must be practised and refined.

The coach is required to have a detailed and up-to-date knowledge of the technical aspects of the sport he or she is coaching so they can feedback any errors in skill execution. Another factor to consider is the production of a clear criterion by which to observe performance. For example, the hockey coach in observing a player moving with the ball would look at the head, body, hand positions on the stick, footwork and ball in that order to identify whether the skill was being executed properly.

To observe effectively the coach must move around the performer or the group in order to view performance from a range of different angles. For example, the gymnastics coach who is observing his or her performer on the asymmetric bars should take positions from the front,

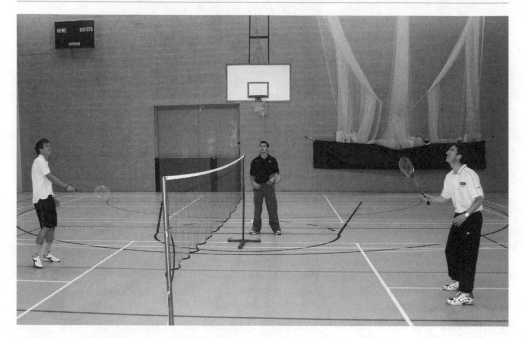

Photo 5.4 A coach observing performance.

back, left and right sides in order to observe the correct form of the movement while the skill is being executed. The coach should also be in a good position to observe the dismount and landing. The coach needs to see the skill performed a number of times in order that a number of observations can be made, leading to an objective assessment of effective or ineffective skill execution by the performer.

McMorris and Hale (2006) suggest that as novice coaches develop the skill of observation they build up a basic model or picture of what the skill should look like. When the coach becomes more expert and attuned to the finer technical detail of their sport, and develops an understanding of the biomechanics of movement, they will be able to observe in more detail the intricacies of movement and consequently be able to make an informed and objective judgement of whether the skill needs to be corrected or not.

For example, the trampoline coach observing a performer who was dropping a shoulder in a front somersault would identify that this could affect the form of the skill in terms of the body being misaligned for the execution of the next part of the routine. Identifying the position of the shoulder is diagnostic observation of a high level that a novice coach might miss, but the expert coach is able to highlight the error because of their experience in knowing what to look for.

Developing the skill (or art) of observation does present difficulties, as in many cases the coach is the only person doing the observing, and this is not the only problem that the coach will face. Crisfield *et al.* (2003) identify the speed of unfolding events, the amount of information the coach can process, perception of events, observational bias, and the blur of action and key events distorting the reliability of information as limiting factors in the observational process.

Many sports are fast-moving and the amount of information presented to the coach to attend to and store for recall is considerable. To be able to effectively recall a whole 90 minutes of soccer action is impossible. Franks and Miller (1986) found that soccer coaches were less than 45 per cent correct in post-game assessment of the first 45 minutes of a soccer game.

Moreover, coaches appear to see things differently, which is due to the different perception and interpretation of unfolding events, and quite often a bias exists which at an unconscious level reduces the accuracy of observation. An example of this would be the coach who, because he or she views a particular player as aesthetically more skilful, might not notice another player who executes the basics very well with no fuss. Events in sport happen very quickly and this blur of action can cause confusion and false impressions, and key events such as officiating decisions can distort the reliability and reality of the recall of what actually occurred.

Fortunately, technology is now readily available to support the coach in developing his or her observational skills. The coach now has at his or her disposal the use of video, DVDs, DV cameras and digital cameras which allow the coach to replay performance repeatedly in order to effectively observe and thus analyse performance. Figure 5.8 shows a model that describes the observation process from the perspective of inputs into the process.

FEEDBACK

In this section feedback will be looked at from a practical perspective, while in Chapter 14 (Skill acquisition and the role of the coach) feedback will be looked at in more detail from a theoretical point of view. Provision of feedback to the performer is a further crucial component in coaching practice.

The performer requires feedback in order to know whether or not they are executing the skill effectively. Feedback must be meaningful to the performer; it is of no use to the performer if the coach says "well done", "excellent", "great skills", "good shot" – the feedback being presented must be specific to the task. The coach needs to tell the performer why they executed a skill well. In soccer, for example, if it was a good shot then the coach should say "That was a good shot, because you had your head over the ball, you were in balance in your approach to the ball and you also hit the ball through the laces".

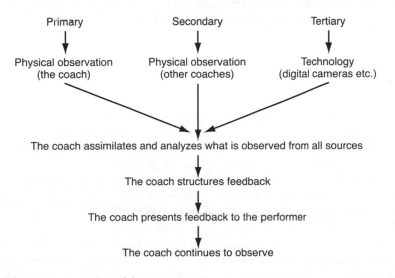

Figure 5.8 Observation process model.

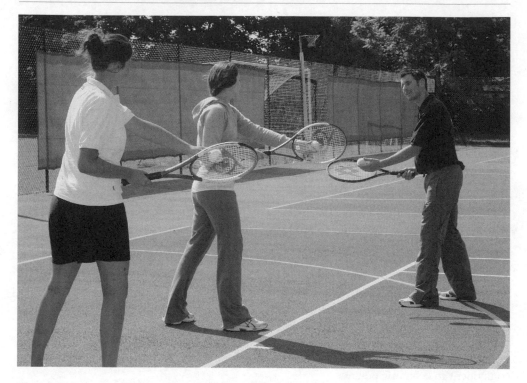

Photo 5.5 A coach correcting errors and providing feedback.

Most GBoS coaching manuals correctly identify that the "sandwich approach" should be taken in providing feedback to performers, which is provision of a positive comment, then a negative and finally another positive one. The coach must also be careful with the amount of feedback they provide the performer. They should not overload the performer with a large amount of verbal information; it should be broken down into bite-size chunks, which is of special importance when working with children. When working with elite performers the feedback provided will be more precise, finer in detail and highly technical.

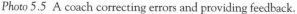

SUMMARY

The coach needs to be aware of their behaviour in certain situations, and how that behaviour can impact upon the performer and the coach-athlete relationship. The coach's leadership style is also of importance because they are in a position that requires decisions to be made, and performers will look to the coach to make those decisions.

The coach should develop a range of coaching styles, which makes for effective coaching, and at the same time they should account for their performers' learning styles. It is useful for the coach to know their own learning style and be aware that if they deliver in their own preferred style, they are not accounting for the needs of all the performers.

The coach has to have an understanding of how to differentiate in order to account for different ability levels in practices, and also how to adapt practices to account for individual and group needs. How the coach communicates either verbally or non-verbally has a significant impact upon coaching delivery, and although a lot of information is provided from a verbal perspective, it is the non-verbal communication that performers pick up on more.

Demonstrations are a key component in coaching delivery and should be provided at the start of practice, during practice and at the end to reinforce the coaching points. The coach needs to practise and refine their observation skills, and have a detailed understanding of their sport's technical requirements. In order to support the observation process the coach has technology at their disposal in the form of video, DVDs and DV cameras.

Finally, the coach is required to give the performer clear and concise feedback in order to improve performance, and as general rule the "sandwich approach" should be used when providing feedback.

SEMINAR OR DISCUSSION QUESTIONS

1. Discuss the differences between reactive and spontaneous behaviours.
2. What would be the impact of the coach staying in his her preferred learning style when delivering a coaching session?
3. What non-verbal communication characteristics might the coach display, and what effect might they have on his or her performers?

KEY TERMS AND DEFINITIONS

- Activist – likes learning by doing.
- Coaching behaviour – the behavioural responses exhibited by the coach in response to his or her performer's behaviour.
- Coaching style – the way in which the coach delivers his or her coaching session.
- Differentiation – changing the practice to account for the ability needs of the individual.
- Demonstration – provision of appropriate visual information for developing a memory template.
- Feedback – meaningful information regarding skill execution provided from either an internal or external source.
- Learning style – the manner and conditions under which learners most efficiently, and effectively perceive, process, store and recall what they are attempting to learn.
- Non-verbal communication – body language.
- Observation – ability to know what to look for in a logical order.
- Pragmatist – likes learning by trying.
- Reactive behaviour – the coach's reaction to the team or performer.
- Reflector – likes learning by discussion.
- Situation-specific or contingency theories – suggest an interaction between the leader and the situation.
- Spontaneous behaviour – initiated by the coach and is not in response to the player's behaviour.
- Theorist – likes learning facts.

- Trait theory – certain leaders have personality traits and personality characteristics that make them ideally suited for leadership.
- Universal behaviours – the idea that successful leaders have certain universal behaviours.
- Verbal communication – instruction.

WEB LINKS

Coaching styles – www.humankinetics.com/SuccessfulCoaching
Self Improvement Association – www.sia-hq.com

FURTHER READING

Cox, R. H. (2007). *Sport Psychology: Concepts and Applications* (6th edn). McGraw-Hill, New York, pp. 306–23.

Foxon, F. (2001). *Improving Practices and Skills*. Coachwise/SportsCoachUK, Leeds.

Horn, T. S. (2008). *Advances in Sport Psychology* (3rd edn). Human Kinetics, Champaign, IL.

Loo, T. (2009). 14 qualities of a true leader. Self-Improvement Associaton (SIA). Online: www.sia-hq.com/articles/14-Qualities-of-a-true-leader (accessed 14th October 2009).

McMorris, T. (2004). *Acquisition and Performance of Sports Skills*. Wiley & Sons, Chichester.

McMorris, T. and Hale, T. (2006). *Coaching Science: Theory into Practice*. Wiley & Sons, Chichester.

Martens, R. (1987). *Coaches Guide to Sport Psychology*. Human Kinetics, Champaign, IL.

Robertson, K. (2002). *Observation, Analysis and Video*. Coachwise/SportsCoachUK, Leeds.

Chapter 6

Structuring practice

CHAPTER OBJECTIVES

- Explain the structure of a coaching session.
- Identify and describe practice principles.
- Explain how to run practices.
- Identify, describe and differentiate between types of practice that are available to the coach.

STRUCTURING A COACHING SESSION

The first step in the coaching process is to plan the session, which involves selecting the technique you want to coach and writing it down on a session plan (planning will be looked at in more detail in Chapter 7). When the coach arrives at the venue they must carry out a health and safety assessment, and set up the practices prior to the performers arriving. Once this has been completed and the performers have arrived, there is a suggested process that the coach should go through, from introduction all the way through to ending the session and self-evaluation.

Chambers (1997) suggests that once you have selected the skill, the keys to effective teaching are the explanation, demonstration, practice, and feedback and error correction. However, this author would argue that the process is a lot more detailed and therefore offers a more comprehensive approach. Once the coach arrives and has the group's attention they should introduce themselves (assuming it is a new group) and go through a health and safety brief which accounts for medical complaints, injuries, jewellery and ensuring the participants are wearing specialist safety equipment. A facility safety brief should also be given. The coach should then instigate the warm-up.

Once the warm-up has been completed the coach should outline the aims and objectives of the session, and how the skill relates to the context of the game or performance. The coach should then demonstrate the skill to be practised, include the coaching points associated with the skill and demonstrate in a position that the group can see and hear effectively. A good strategy would be organizing the group into a semi-circle in order that everyone can see the demonstration. This should be quite brief because the coach should ensure that the players then get the opportunity to practise the skill. While the group are practising the skill, the coach should move around the group observing and analysing performance.

If required, the coach should step in and offer corrective feedback on an individual basis

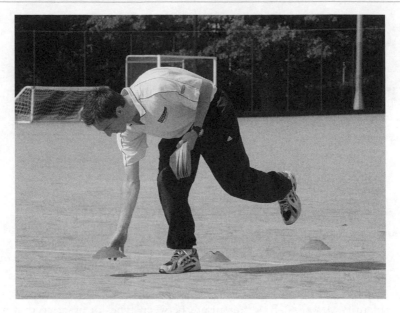

Photo 6.1 A coach setting up a practice.

in order to improve performance. If the coach feels that the whole group is struggling in executing the skill they should call the group in for group feedback, revisit the demonstration and reinforce the key coaching points. Using a question and answer strategy during this group feedback session is also useful in testing the performers' understanding. The performers should then be allowed to practise.

If the performers have managed to execute the skill effectively, then the coach should move on to the next progression. This again would involve calling the group back in, offering a demonstration with the key coaching points and providing the opportunity to practise as soon as possible. The corrective feedback process is then repeated in order to account for individual and group needs and to improve performance. The coach may go through two, three or four progressions depending on the length of the session and the performers' ability to learn what is being delivered to them.

The end product of the session should involve (if in a team game) a game-related scenario which puts the skill being learnt into the context of the game. This can be achieved by using small-sided games, tactical situations or game play with task constraints included. The session should be concluded with a cool-down. While the cool-down is being completed it provides the opportunity for the coach to clear away the equipment.

The final part of the process is the coach self-evaluating his or her performance and carrying out a post-practice feedback session with the group. This provides the coach with the opportunity to ask the performers questions regarding the key coaching points of the skills they have learnt to test their understanding. Once this has been completed the coach should look forward to the next coaching session and let the performers know briefly what will be covered.

This process may be viewed as rather a mechanistic way of approaching coaching practice but the components outlined are key ingredients in the routine delivery of coaching practice. There are of course slight variations in the ways that practices can be set up, e.g. whole-part-whole (see below), but they all contain basically the same ingredients.

PRINCIPLES OF PRACTICE

Coaching sessions provide the athlete with the perfect environment in which to learn new skills and techniques. Coaches should plan and construct progressive coaching practices that provide a challenging environment and allow performers to acquire, apply and execute a range of techniques in training and competition (Foxon, 2001).

One of the fundamental aims of practice is identifying the needs of the performer or performers, and having a plan to facilitate these needs. The coach needs to outline the aims and objectives of the session because the performers will want to know what they are doing and why they are doing it. Keeping the length of practice on time is a key principle, and the coach will need to plan enough practices to fulfil the needs of the individual or the group, and at the same time keep within the allotted time allowed for the practice.

There are two scenarios that do not lend itself to good practice. One is the coach completing the practice schedule far too early and not having enough practices planned, consequently the session runs out of steam. In the other scenario the coach spends far too much time on a practice and runs out of time. However, situations do arise when either the coach is unable to progress the performers fluidly, or the performers grasp what is being delivered quicker than expected. In these situations flexibility in the planning process (having a contingency plan) would be appropriate, and the ability to adapt within the session is crucial. The coach should also prioritize practices that they intend to cover over a period of time, which can be integrated into the overall season plan (season planning is discussed in Chapter 8).

The coach should keep the practice active and organize the practice session so that queues do not build up on cones. In team sports, if the coach allows queues to build up it can affect the fluency of the session; the intensity at which the performers are working at because they are standing and waiting in turn for their practice; their motivation because their needs may not being fulfilled; and on a cold night the performers will get cold, which increases the risk of injury. A further consideration is that when a particular skill is being delivered it must be put into a game-related practice at some point in the session so that the performer can put the skill and practice into the context of the game.

The coach should also take into account the length of time they take delivering a repetitive practice. Do not "drill for drilling's sake" as it can become de-motivational. If the coach does intend to use this principle to reinforce a particular skill, they should at least vary the practice schedule, at the same time maintaining the skill theme.

RUNNING PRACTICES

Hinkson (2001) suggest that when running the practice it should be broken into four parts: physical conditioning, skill practices (technical development), team practices (tactical development) and mental preparation. The coach can incorporate physical conditioning into many if not all of their practices. For example, the netball coach may introduce a high intensity chest passing exercise that only gives the players a short recovery time (5 seconds) between cones or practice stations, and the coach may keep this up for a period of time in order to develop aerobic and anaerobic capacity.

Speed, Agility and Quickness (SAQ®) principles are now being implemented in a range of sports such as soccer, rugby, hockey, cricket, tennis and golf (SAQ®, 2008). SAQ® training develops fundamental movement skills and physical conditioning using ladders and hurdles (SAQ®, 2003). With imagination the coach can use a variety of equipment that focuses on components of fitness and integrate this into skill development at the same time. Doing this has a number of benefits: it improves fitness; makes fitness sessions more fun and interesting for the performer; and it helps develop coordination of the skill with coordination of body movement more effectively.

The second element of running a practice should include development of core skills that make up the basics of the game. The basics should be practised well so that they can be executed without conscious thought. At times during the season (and practice) the coach will need to break down these skills into their component parts and revisit them in order to reinforce effective learning.

The third element of running a practice comprises of tactical development (working with a team) or development of a complete performance routine (working with an individual). The volley ball coach may have been working on a specific set and spike routine in isolation, but in order for it to be fully effective it should be integrated into a full game situation and practised as a specific tactic. In an individual performance environment the high jump coach may work on the approach to the high jump in isolation to get the footwork right in order for the take-off to be executed effectively. The coach would then put the whole routine of approach, take off, clearing the bar and landing together as a complete performance.

The final element of running a practice is the inclusion of mental skills training. Types of mental skills that the coach may integrate into their coaching include goal setting, imagery, concentration techniques, confidence enhancement, development of pre-performance and pre-competition routines, and anxiety reduction and/or inducement. Mental skills, like motor skills, do take time to practise, and integration of them into practice sessions can be more effective than if they are delivered in isolation. A more detailed outline of mental skills training and the coach is explored in Chapter 13.

The coach should plan well and also have a contingency plan to account for the unexpected. If the soccer coach plans for 12 players and three goalkeepers to conduct a shooting and goalkeeping session, and only eight players and no goalkeepers turn up, then a contingency plan would not be remiss. To be fully effective in running a practice the coach should not participate with the performers. The reasons for this are that the coach is unable to observe effectively and therefore unable to offer feedback on performance; it takes practice time away from the performers; it interferes with the task that is being delivered; and, as Hinkson (2001) argues, coaches are more credible if they provide verbal information rather than showing how they can play the game.

Quality rather than quantity of practice should be a major focus for the coach when delivering a coaching session, and different exercises should be implemented that are practised at game or performance pace. Hinkson (2001) further suggests that the coach should avoid too much repetition, always look for improvement, introduce new skills early and not condone or accept bad habits.

TYPES OF PRACTICE

Practice is essential if learning is to take place (McMorris and Hale, 2006), and deciding on which type of practice to deliver the session with will depend on how and what the coach requires his or her performers to learn. There are other factors that may influence this decision. Is the skill being coached best delivered in parts? Does the coach have enough time to spend on developing a series of progressions or is there time to spend on the whole practice?

An example of delivering the whole practice would be the triple jump coach coaching the whole routine from the approach run to the hop, step and jump and landing. The coach however does need to consider the ability of the group if he or she is delivering a session in the whole mode. If, for example, the coach is coaching a beginner the triple jump, the beginner will be limited in their full understanding of the technical requirements of the task, because of the amount of information that they may have to attend to in performing the task. This applies to many sports so the coach therefore needs to consider how he or she structures practice for the beginner.

If the coach decides that the most effective delivery mode is in parts, they will divide the technique into its component parts and instruct the performer to practise it separately. The part delivery mode can be structured in two ways: the part-progressive practice and the part-continuous practice. The part-progressive practice is where each component is practised in isolation before being recombined and practised together (Foxon, 2001).

For example, the surfing coach delivering dry-land drills before going out on the water would coach the skills of the paddling stroke, pushing the arms up to bring the legs through the body in order to stand up, then adjusting body and feet to effectively balance on the board separately, before recombining the three elements. The part-continuous practice is where each component is introduced in a continuous and progressive logical sequence so that they all gradually build up to form the whole technique (Foxon, 2001). The surfing coach would first coach the paddling stroke, then the paddling stroke and pushing the arms up to bring the legs through the body to stand up, and finally paddling, pushing the arms up to bring the legs through the body to stand up and adjusting feet and body all together.

In teams sports quite often a sequential series of progressions is used, which is a progression of overload situations leading into a tactical or game play. For example, in rugby, soccer, hockey or basketball the coach may start with a 1 v. 1 practice then progress to a 2 v. 1, 2 v. 2, 3 v. 2 and 3 v. 3, with the final progression being a tactical situation or a full game. This type of sequential progression is useful for developing skill and decision-making qualities in performers. Hinkson (2001) argues that drills have to be progressive so that players get the feeling of success. If the performers are not achieving success with the 3 v. 2 practice then the coach can "regress" to a 3 v. 1 or further down to a 3 v. 0, in order to achieve success.

This process of regression for progression is another useful strategy in manipulating and enhancing the decision-making processes in the performer. A range of team sports progressions can also be developed using resistance, in which passive and active defenders or attackers can be used to add or decrease pressure and decision making. Space can also be used as a progression in terms of reducing the size of the practice area, which increases the pressure on the performer.

Whole-part-whole is another type of practice that is available to the coach. The coach presents the whole practice and the practice is then broken down into its component parts, and then the whole is practised again in order to see if effective learning of the parts has taken place. Whole-part-whole is not just game, skill, game. In a team sport the whole can comprise a tactical element, the part the practising of a skill within that tactical element and then re-introducing the tactical element as the whole. Another example would be the surfer on his or her dry-land drills practising the whole skill of getting up on the surf board. They would practice the whole routine first, and then practice pushing the arms up to bring the legs through the body to stand up, and finally back to practising the whole routine.

SUMMARY

Coaching sessions provide the athlete with the perfect environment in which to learn new skills and techniques. In order to facilitate this, the coach needs to consider a range of issues when structuring practice sessions. Chambers (1997) provides a basic framework to explain how a session should be structured, which includes explanation, demonstration, practice, and feedback and correction. However, this author has suggested a more detailed and comprehensive approach. There are certain factors that the coach should consider in structuring practice and these include having a plan, identifying the needs of the individual, outlining aims and objectives, keeping on time, prioritizing the practices that are to be delivered and putting the skills practised into a game or performance-related context. Hinkson (2001) identifies that the practice should be broken down into four distinct parts, the physical conditioning, technical delivery, team or tactical delivery and mental preparation.

The coach in the planning stage of writing his or her session plan should account for all these components and, after a period of time, integration of these four core components will become second nature to the practising coach. Practice is essential if learning is to take place (McMorris and Hale, 2006), and deciding on which type of practice to deliver in the session will depend on how and what the coach requires his or her performers to learn. The coach should ask themselves whether the skill being coached is best delivered in parts and whether there is enough time to spend on developing a series of progressions or enough time to spend on the whole practice. Different practice types exist, which include whole practice, part practice (which is either delivered in a part-progressive or part-continuous mode), whole-part-whole or the sequential progression method, which predominantly lends itself to team sports.

SEMINAR OR DISCUSSION QUESTIONS

1. Structure a practice in a sport of your choice utilizing Hinkson's (2001) suggested four components of practice.
2. Construct a part-progressive, part-continuous, whole-part-whole and a sequential progression practice in a sport of your choice.

KEY TERMS AND DEFINITIONS

-   Part-continuous practice – each component is introduced in a continuous and progressive logical sequence so that they all gradually build up to form the whole technique.
-   Part-progressive – each component is practised in isolation before being recombined and practised together.
-   SAQ® Speed, Agility and Quickness – a concept that focuses on developing fundamental motor abilities, agility, balance and coordination.
-   Sequential progression – a progression of overload situations leading into a tactical or game play.

- Type of practice – a method of practice delivery.
- Whole-part-whole – the coach presents the whole practice, then the practice is broken down into its component parts, then the whole is practised again.

WEB LINKS

SAQ® – www.saqinternational.com

FURTHER READING

Chambers, D. (1997). *Coaching: The Art and the Science*. Key Porter, Toronto.
Foxon, F. (2001). *Improving Practices and Skills*. Coachwise/SportsCoachUK, Leeds.
Hinkson, J (2001). *The Art of Team Coaching*. Warwick Publishing, Toronto.
McMorris, T. and Hale. T. (2006). *Coaching Science: Theory into Practice*. Wiley & Sons, Chichester.

Planning, management and the role of the coach

INTRODUCTION

Part 3 outlines the planning process from a micro (session plan) to a macro (season plan) perspective and also considers the coach in a management role. Chapter 7 explains why the coach should plan a coaching session, and describes the Plan, Lead, Reflect process, which is also known as the Plan, Conduct, Evaluate or Plan, Do, Review process. An explanation of how the coach should construct a session plan is provided, together with the core elements that should be contained within the plan. The coach's role in the self-reflection and evaluation process is discussed, and points that the coach should consider in the evaluation process are listed.

Chapter 7 explains how block planners (meso cycles) are constructed and how they fit into the planning process. Case studies of how coaches in different sports approach their planning of coaching sessions are also a feature of this chapter. Chapter 7 is supported by the provision of appendices (at the end of the book) that include examples of a practice needs analysis, a session plan, a block planner and an evaluation.

Chapter 8 focuses on season planning and the long-term planning process, and identifies the core components of a season plan. The process of carrying out a performance requirement analysis is explained, with an example provided in the appendices. Chapter 8 also explains the process of periodization, individualization and peaking and tapering. These concepts are core elements in the long-term planning process, which the coach should have a good working knowledge of.

Chapter 9 explores the role of the coach as a manager, and the issues that are associated with managing people. Basic management theory will be identified and explained from the early classical movement of management theory to the more contemporary total quality management perspective, which is presented as a fundamentally better way to manage. Human resource management is explained as a concept and applied in the coaching context, with examples provided of a coach having senior management roles and responsibilities. Chapter 9 also identifies specific management roles that the coach may have to fulfil, as quite often the coach is working in isolation, and therefore finds him or herself in a multi-role capacity. A comparison is made of the North American coaching system with the UK amateur and professional club system. This chapter highlights how best the coach can manage the coaching environment, and its final section explores issues of conflict and the role of the coach, and how best to resolve conflict. At the end of each chapter seminar or discussion questions and key terms and definitions are provided to support student learning. Web links and further reading are also provided in order for the student to carry out continued research if required.

Chapter 7

Planning a coaching session

CHAPTER OBJECTIVES

- Explain why a coach should plan.
- Explain the Plan, Lead, Reflect process.
- Describe how session plans are constructed.
- Highlight the process of self-reflection, the purpose of evaluations and how the coach should construct an evaluation.
- Describe why block planners are used and how to construct them.
- Provide a case study of how a soccer coach plans for a coaching session.
- Provide a case study of how a netball coach plans for a coaching session.

WHY A COACH SHOULD PLAN

Arguably, planning is the most important element in the coaching process. Coaching sessions need to be planned to help performers achieve short-, medium- and long-term goals, which influence the content, duration, intensity and structure of the session (Foxon, 2001). Crisfield et al. (2003) further suggest that effective plans should be structured to meet the needs of the individual or team, contain specific challenging goals and be adaptable to achieve the practice aims and objectives.

A session plan is an organized scheme of work that allows the coach to deliver, monitor and assess specific aims and objectives of practice. The planning process should start a long time before the season or performance starts, and the coach will need to gather certain pieces of information to fulfil the planning process before they conduct the session. A practice needs analysis (see Appendix 4) can be used in order for the coach to identify and account for certain needs in the planning process, such as:

- who the group are
- previous experience and ability
- individual needs
- how many players
- age of players (junior or adult)
- gender
- session aims and objectives
- length of session

- venue
- facility and equipment needs
- medical information
- health and safety issues
- availability of support staff.

(Robinson, 2006b)

Once this information has been collected by the coach they are in a better position to start putting a session plan together because they have specific information to start setting goals for the performers and account for individual and group needs. Hinkson (2001) suggests that practices are almost as important as games, and that coaches have to be organized in practice because most of their work is done there. Without a plan, it is difficult to identify the starting and finishing points or the best route between the two, and there will be no real focus in a coaching session, which can impact upon the athletes motivation and sense of achievement (Crisfield *et al.*, 2003). Bearing this statement in mind, planning is an integral element of the coaching process, and considered, effective and detailed planning should not be understated.

PLAN, LEAD, REFLECT

Plan, Do, Review; Plan, Practice, Reflect; Plan, Lead, Evaluate; Plan, Conduct, Evaluate or Plan, Lead, Reflect – the coach will see all of these in books that try to explain the overall coaching process. They all basically mean the same and are interchangeable – the coach can use anyone of them to explain the coaching process. For the purpose of this section Plan, Lead, Reflect will be used to explain the basic principles behind the coaching process. The coaching delivery is determined by the three core elements of Plan, Lead and Reflect.

1. Plan – planning is essential; the plan should be flexible and have a contingency; it should identify and account for every performer's needs; enough practices within the session should be planned to fulfil the aims and objectives and account for performer needs; health and safety must also be accounted for.
2. Lead – leading the session, which should include a warm-up, instruction, demonstrations, observation, error correction, feedback, practice, progression, motivation, cool-down.
3. Reflect – reflecting on, reviewing and evaluating what went well, what did not go so well, how the session could have been improved and how to action plan suggested improvements.

Figure 7.1 shows a pictorial representation of the Coaching Process Cycle. This is a very simple way of looking at the coaching process, but it is what the coach should be aiming for at the very least. When the coach is in the early stages of their coaching career, planning is very basic, which is to be expected and Jones *et al.* (1997) reinforce this statement by stating that "novice coaches do not plan as well as more experienced coaches". However, as the coach develops, gains experience and progresses through his or her GBoS Coach Awards, planning should become more considered and detailed.

If the coach is working with a group of coaches, the senior coach should construct the overall plan, but with input from the other coaches. During the lead phase of the process the senior coach should delegate certain elements of the plan to the support coaches to deliver,

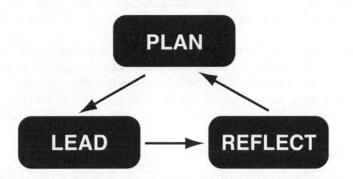

Figure 7.1 Coaching Process Tri-Cycle.

and should oversee the overall session supporting and providing input when required. When reflecting, all the coaches should be engaged in this process in order to evaluate the session effectively.

CONSTRUCTION OF SESSION PLANS

The previous two sections explained why the coach should plan and the nature of the coaching process; this section will identify how the session plan itself should be constructed. A range of different session plans exist, but they all contain certain basic elements. A session may run for one hour, one-and-a-half hours, two hours or sometimes longer and the coach will therefore need to plan according to the time available.

An example of a session plan for a field hockey practice session lasting one-and-a-half hours is shown in Appendix 5. Once all the relevant information is gathered the coach needs to sit down and construct the plan on paper or use a computer spreadsheet to record the information, which many coaches find easier than physically writing it out. Also, there are website addresses and companies that offer already constructed practices online for a range of sports. At the top of the session plan the following basic headings should be present:

- the team, club or performer being coached
- the date of the session
- the session number
- the session aims and objectives
- the number of participants
- the ability of the group
- the resources required to coach the session (balls, cones, bibs, etc.).

The plan should have a column down one side that outlines the timings and themes of the session. At the very least, the principle themes should include the warm-up, an introductory session (which may be revisiting a skill from the previous week), a skills section, a tactical or modified games section (assuming the coach is working with a team) and finally a section for the cool-down. A second column to the right of the first column should then detail the content of each of the principal themes in terms of coaching points, progressions, organization of practices and small diagrams. On the back of the session plan there should be a section for an evaluation and, ideally, the risk assessment for the facility should also be attached to the plan.

As the coach becomes more experienced and the level of planning becomes more detailed, then the elements that make up the session plan should become more expansive. For example, a section covering individual needs (players returning from injury), physiological and psychological components, organization and management (utilization of support staff) and how the session is going to account for differentiation may also be included.

REFLECTION AND EVALUATION

Reflection is a multi-faceted and complex process that is instrumental in supporting effective coaching in terms of evaluation and good practice, and is essential for the coach's development. Ghaye (2001) highlights that four guiding principles underpin reflective practice: it is about the coach and his or her practice; it is about learning from experience; it is about valuing what you do and why you do it; the reflective conversation is pivotal to reflecting.

Self-reflection is also central to the evaluation process. Constructing the post-session or post-season evaluation; developing the ability to self-reflect; and reviewing and evaluating coaching performance are all parts of an ongoing and continually learnt process. Evaluation drives change for the next coaching session or series of sessions and must be constructed in a meaningful way.

However, the coach should be careful about when they actually evaluate the session. Although the coach should reflect upon the session straight away and involve other coaches and players, it is recommended that they should not actually write up their evaluation until a couple days after the session. The primary reason for this is that a major event, such as conflict between the coach and performer(s), could have impacted upon the outcome of the session. Therefore, it is better to reflect fully and then write up the evaluation when the coach is more able to have a clear and objective perspective of events.

The coach should consider the following points when evaluating a coaching session. This is not an exhaustive list and serves only as a suggested guide, as there are a range of factors that can impact upon the delivery of a coaching session. An example of an evaluation is shown in Appendix 6.

- Were the practice aims and objectives achieved?
- Was the content appropriate to the needs of the participants?
- Were the resources adequate and appropriate?
- Were correct and sufficient coaching points provided?
- Were there suitable progressions and were they pitched at the right level?
- Did the coach observe, analyse and monitor performance effectively?
- Was feedback provided in a timely and effective fashion, to both the individual and group?
- Was feedback gained from the participants at key points during the session?
- Was feedback gained from others (coaches, managers and support staff)?
- Were the coaching style and communication appropriate?
- Did the coach abide by the Code of Conduct for Sports Coaches?
- Was health and safety accounted for?
- What changes are required for the session?
- What changes are required for the next planned session?

CONSTRUCTION AND USE OF BLOCK PLANNERS

A block planner is a scheme of work that highlights general aims and objectives over an extended cycle from which the session plans are derived. Generally, the block planner consists of a four–six week block of work (also known as a meso cycle). The sessions contained within the block planner must show a clear progression of technique and tactics for a team sport, or skill development over a period of time for an individual sport. Block planners should contain the following information:

- session aims and objectives
- appropriate technical content
- appropriate tactical development (if working with a team)
- appropriate progressions
- fitness components to be worked on.

(Robinson, 2006b)

An example block planner of a trampoline coach's scheme of work for four weeks is given in Appendix 7. As with session plans, the block planner must be evaluated at the end of the cycle. Although the planning process is an integral part of the coaching process, different coaches approach the process in different ways, and flexibility is often highlighted as a significant factor in the way that they plan. The following case studies are of a male and female coach respectively in two very different sports who provide different perspectives in the way they approach the planning process.

Case study 7.1 – The soccer coach and planning

Jordan has been coaching for six years and is a Level 2 soccer coach who is currently coaching at an English Premiership soccer club Junior Development Centre. Jordan is an organized coach who plans for every one of his coaching sessions, and takes at least 20 minutes to write out the overall plan. Within his session plan Jordan highlights an overall aim for the session, with objectives to be met as the session progresses. He also includes a detailed warm-up and constructs a series of progressions that lead into a modified game.

Jordan ensures that a contingency plan is also included to account for any change in the group size or if any of the session objectives are not being met. Accounting for differentiation forms a large part in the planning process because of the large range of abilities that are present at the Junior Development Centre. Although Jordan has not used a practice needs analysis for this particular group, he has used a performance profile. He has utilized the performance profile to evaluate the players' ability at the start of the season, so that he can monitor and assess their progress in training.

A range of sources are used to provide ideas on how to construct practices, which include in-house handbooks with practices already constructed. Jordan also observes other coaches, which gives him ideas of types of practices he can construct. He does not use websites or electronic sources to print his plans out because he feels writing them out is more personalized and therefore better. Jordan keeps all his session plans and shares them with other coaches, which he feels that every coach should do because comparing thoughts and ideas can improve coaching practice.

As well as coaching at the Junior Development Centre, Jordan also coaches at residential camps. When putting his session plans together for the residential camps he ensures that they are a lot more detailed than the ones he produces for the Junior Development Centre. At the residential camps there are a lot of senior professional coaches, and Jordan wants to ensure that these coaches are aware of the level of planning that he puts into his coaching, and also that he is working at a professional level. This is not to say that his planning is any less detailed when coaching at the Junior Development Centre; his plans still contain the necessary information for him and his assistant to professionally and effectively deliver the session.

There is a specific type of session plan that Jordan uses which is provided by the GBoS, however, it does not allow for much detail and he is not sure how many coaches actually use them. Jordan considers himself to be a very organized coach and he ensures that the session is set up before the group arrives. He feels that players appreciate this, and they tend to focus early on in the exercises rather than waiting around for the coach to set the practices up. Being organized shows a high degree of professionalism, which helps the players feel that they are involved in a professional environment.

Another aspect of Jordan's planning involves the use of block planners, which are constructed for a four–six week period, and they have been integrated into his coaching practice because of the knowledge he gained about how to plan effectively while studying a Sports Coaching Science degree at university.

At the end of every session Jordan goes through the evaluation process, which also involves his assistant coach, and between them they highlight the strengths and weaknesses of the session and subsequently how they could improve it. In going through this process he feels that he has developed the ability to self-reflect at a considered level. However, he does feel that he would like to have the opportunity to share his reflections with a senior coach, and he feels uncomfortable with the fact that there is no system in place in his present position to enable this. Jordan feels he needs someone to positively criticize and have input into his coaching session, as he needs feedback on his coaching performance – otherwise he doesn't know whether he is improving or not. He suggested it would be good to have a role model or mentor system in place like other sports, because it would provide him with the opportunity to fully reflect upon his own coaching experience.

Case study 7.2 – The netball coach and planning

Jane is an All England Netball Association educator and tutor for UKCC Levels 1, 2 and 3, and an assessor. She is also a British Association of Sport and Exercise Science accredited sport psychologist (sports science support). Jane has been coaching for over 20 years, and has coached the English and British Universities netball team and is involved with the Brunel London Talent League.

Jane always plans her sessions but not always in a specific format, and a contingency plan is developed to account for any eventuality in her coaching, because the coaching environment she is in demands a high degree of flexibility. A lot of time is spent on planning, and thinking about planning, and Jane has two methods that she uses. When she is coaching on her own she takes around two hours to construct a session plan, but when she is coaching with a team of coaches this process can take longer. When working with a team of assistant coaches Jane is on the phone discussing and exchanging ideas. If she is working with senior coaches she sends out emails so that suggested comments and areas of adaptation can be identified and discussed. Jane does not write so much detail into her plans now as she did when she first started out coaching, because she feels that she is more experienced now. However, she always has a focus on the outcomes of the session, what the last activity requires the players to do, and ensures that the session is progressive.

A practice needs analysis is not used in a formal way, but Jane observes a new group play, how they structure combinations, their body management and ball work, and she also asks players about themselves, in terms of what their needs are and what they want to achieve. Sometimes emails are sent to players to ask them how they want the session structured, which Jane feels engages the player in the whole plan.

A plan is physically written for every session and a file is kept, so that it can be a reference to restructure previous ideas for new groups. Jane believes that website practices are limited because physically writing out a session plan fully engages the coach in the planning process. Jane produces detailed or rough-guide session plans, and this will depend on who she is working with. If she is coaching on her own she will produce a rough guide, confident that she is knowledgeable enough to deliver the coaching points accurately. However, if she is working with other coaches she will produce a more detailed plan. She might not always follow the format, as often she needs to adapt to unexpected changes in the environment. Jane adapts the session plan format available through the GBoS to suit the needs of the situation. However, she does feel that the format is useful for new coaches starting out because it is not easy to use.

Block planning does not always feature in the planning process for Jane, however, she does look at players and identify the cycle of planning they are in, and at cycles used by other coaches. During the summer Jane constructs training programmes for individuals, and she feels that it is important that you plan and that the players see that you plan well because it provides a process by which the coach knows where they are going with a session. Moreover, she feels that you must have structure in your planning in order to be able to adapt.

Jane spends long hours agonizing about and reflecting upon her coaching sessions and spends a lot of time discussing evaluations with other coaches. She goes through a long reflection process, especially after a match. Players are also included in the evaluation and reflection process, and feedback is always asked of the players to improve the delivery of the next coaching session. Jane does not always formally write out her evaluations, but she always spends time consciously reflecting on her performance as a coach, and she is happy to engage in discussion with other coaches to continue to develop her range and depth of ideas.

SUMMARY

Planning is arguably the most important process in coaching practice, and coaching sessions need to be planned to help performers achieve their goals (Foxon, 2001). A session plan is an organized scheme of work that allows the coach to deliver, monitor and assess specific aims and objectives of practice. Before a plan is put together the coach should conduct a practice needs analysis in order to gain information on the group they are coaching. Without a plan, it is difficult to identify the starting and finishing points or the best route between the two (Crisfield et al., 2003). Bearing this statement in mind, planning is an integral element in the coaching process and the importance of considered, effective and detailed planning should not be understated.

Three core elements make up the coaching process – Plan, Lead, Reflect – and it is essential that the coach follows this process every time they organize a coaching session. There a key elements that go into the construction of a session plan and although planning in the initial stages of a coach's career will be basic, as they progress in their career it should become a lot more detailed. Evaluation is a key component in the coaching process and developing the ability to self-reflect, review and evaluate coaching performance is an ongoing and continually learnt process. Evaluation drives change for the next coaching session or series of sessions, and must be constructed in a meaningful way.

Finally, construction of block planners is a core aspect of the planning process. The block planner is a scheme of work that highlights general aims and objectives over an extended cycle, which the session plans are derived from. Generally, the block planner consists of a four–six week block of work, and is known as a meso cycle.

SEMINAR OR DISCUSSION QUESTIONS

1. Explain the purpose of writing a session plan, block planner and evaluation.
2. Identify and describe the core elements of a practice needs analysis.

KEY TERMS AND DEFINITIONS

■ Block planner – a scheme of work that highlights general aims and objectives over an extended cycle which the session plans are derived from.
■ Coaching process – a means by which coaching delivery is determined by the three core elements of Plan, Lead, Reflect.
■ Evaluation – a process by which the coach highlights strengths and weaknesses and how they could improve a coaching session.
■ Practice needs analysis – a process used in order for the coach to gather information to identify and account for certain needs in the planning process.
■ Reflect – to review and evaluate coaching performance.
■ Session plan – an organized scheme of work that allows the coach to deliver, monitor and assess specific aims and objectives of practice.

WEB LINKS

Online practice website – www.sportplan.com
Use a search engine and type in "online sports coaching drills" and a range of websites will be found detailing practices and drills in a range of sports.

FURTHER READING

Crisfield, P., Cabral, P. and Carpenter, F. (2003). *The Successful Coach: Guidelines for Coaching Practice.* Coachwise/SportsCoachUK, Leeds.
Foxon, F. (2001). *Improving Practices and Skills.* Coachwise/SportsCoachUK, Leeds.
Hinkson, J. (2001). *The Art of Team Coaching.* Warwick Publishing, Toronto.
Lyle, J. (2002). *Sports Coaching Concepts: A Framework for Coaches' Behaviour.* Routledge, London.

Chapter 8

Season planning

CHAPTER OBJECTIVES

- Outline the purpose a season plan.
- Identify and describe the contents of a season plan.
- Explain periodization.
- Explain individualization.
- Explain peaking and tapering.

PURPOSE OF A SEASON PLAN

Chapter 7 outlined and explained planning from a short- and medium-term perspective, but the coach also has to consider planning for a longer time period. Season planning is an integral feature of any coach's work, and should form the basis from which to facilitate and enhance performance throughout the season and beyond (Robinson, 2005). Bompa (1994) suggests that the planning process is a structured, methodical, scientific procedure to help athletes achieve optimal levels of training effectiveness and performance.

In the high performance coaching environment long-term training programmes and plans are constructed to account for different cycles in training and competition. For example, the athletics coach may develop a training programme for the track athlete based on a quadrennial (four-year) training cycle to prepare for the Olympics, a biennial (two-year) training cycle to prepare for the World Championships or an annual (one-year) cycle for national championships and any other qualifying competitions that may be entered.

Developing and implementing long-term programmes is not exclusive to the high performance environment; long-term planning should also be implemented at all levels if the coach is to get the best out of his or her performer(s). There are a number of reasons why a season plan should be developed and implemented:

- To identify where the performers(s) are right now in terms of the technical ability, tactical knowledge, fitness and psychological needs.
- To identify the short-, medium- and long-term goals of the performer(s) and coach.
- To provide a season plan that gives the coach and performer(s) a structured route and time-frame by which to achieve the identified goals.

■ To provide a monitoring and evaluation process by which to review the progress of the performer(s) and to adapt the season plan accordingly.

(Adapted from Crisfield *et al.*, 2003 and Galvin and Ledger, 1998)

A season plan can also be influenced by a SWOT (Strengths, Weaknesses, Opportunities and Threats) analysis (Robinson, 2005). For example, the volleyball coach in looking back at the previous season's performance statistics may identify that the percentage of successful service returns was low. As an area of perceived weakness, it could be something for the coach to focus on early in the new season and be part of ongoing technical development for the team.

A SWOT analysis can be also conducted on opponents, providing the coach with information to develop strategies and counter-strategies. For example, the table tennis coach may identify that a future table tennis opponent poses a threat in their ability to disguise the delivery of the ball on a service return. The coach may then plan a series of technical and tactical sessions for his table tennis player to negate the threat of the opponent(s).

CONTENTS OF A SEASON PLAN

Once the coach has decided on the length of the training programme, and has carried out a SWOT analysis, they then need to consider the length of the season – when the season starts and finishes and whether there is a pre-season and if so, when it starts (Crisfield *et al.*, 2003). The coach will have to consider if there are any breaks in the season. For example, the English Soccer Premiership teams can have either a one- or two-week break because of their international players being involved in European or World Cup qualifying matches. Using the same example, the coach would also want to know when these competition periods are in order to structure his or her season plan accordingly and also when the off-season is, in order to factor in rest and recovery periods after a long and strenuous season.

After the coach has an understanding of the time-frames involved in their plan they will need to consider how much time the performer(s) can spend on training. If it is only one night a week then the coach is going to be limited, but if the performer(s) can spend more time training then the coach needs to plan accordingly. Availability of resources in terms of facilities, equipment and support staff will also come into the equation. If the training facility is only available once a week and the performer(s) are available to train twice a week then another facility will be required.

When constructing a season plan the coach should have a good understanding of the demands of the sport they are coaching. In order to identify these demands a performance requirement analysis of the four core components (technical, tactical, physical and psychological) can be carried out so that they can be fully integrated into the season plan. For example, the boxing coach would meet with their boxer at the start of the season and identify which weight the boxer wants to compete at, which in turn would inform any weight management issues that need to be addressed in the overall season plan. The coach would then identify the order of importance of the four core components, which might be in this case physical, technical, tactical and psychological, and then set out developing and implementing the plan accordingly for the boxer. An example of a performance requirement analysis for a boxer is shown in Appendix 8.

PERIODIZATION

Once the coach has identified, collected and collated all the required information to put into the season plan, the next stage of the process is to divide the programme up into distinct training periods. "Each of these [periods] will have different goals and training methods, and are designed to maximize gains in the different components of performance and this process is called periodization" (Galvin and Ledger, 1998, p. 55).

The distinct training periods are called macro, meso and micro cycles. A macro cycle can be a prolonged period of time, dependent on the sport and competitions entered, and can be anything from a few months to several months; a meso cycle is a sub-cycle of the macro cycle and is two–six weeks in duration; the micro cycle is a sub-cycle of the meso cycle and is a training period of two–ten days, with training units (individual practice sessions) incorporated into the micro cycles (Galvin and Ledger, 1998). If, for example, the micro cycle duration is one week, and there are two training sessions in that week, the coach would construct two session plans for that micro cycle.

However, confusion arises when Bompa (1994, p. 185) proposes "a macro cycle represents a phase two to six weeks long", does not recognize meso cycles and identifies micro cycles as having a direct link with macro cycles. This author acknowledges both Bompa and Galvin and Ledger's perspectives, but at the same time offers a simpler solution for coaches who will only be planning over a single season in the UK. If the coach requires more depth of understanding of training methodology and periodization principles, Bompa (1994, 1999) and Galvin and Ledger (1998) provide a comprehensive and detailed analysis of the concepts and processes involved.

Although it is acknowledged that season plans should allow for a degree of flexibility, they also should be structured in a logical, integrated and easy-to-understand fashion, and meet the needs and aspirations of the performer. To this end this author suggests that a macro cycle duration should be 12–16 weeks, a meso cycle four–six weeks (which easily equates to the suggested length of a block planner) and a micro cycle one week. For example, in a 12-week macro cycle the coach is able to construct two 6-week meso cycles, and in each meso cycle six 1-week micro cycles, with one or more training units (training sessions) planned for each micro cycle. In a 16-week macro cycle the coach is able to construct four 4-week meso cycles and four subsequent one-week micro cycles, with one or more training units in each micro cycle. The structuring of three-month (12-week) or four-month (16-week) macro cycles fits nicely into many of the UK domestic sports seasons. This may be viewed as rather a rigid perspective on periodization planning, but the training periods (macro, meso and micro cycles) all dovetail neatly into one another and the process is simplified for the coach who may be constructing their first season plan. It is acknowledged that in implementing either a 4 × 12 or 3 × 16-week macro structure equates to 48 weeks in a 52-week year, so therefore a degree of flexibility in planning should be allowed to take the four-week difference between the season plan and the chronological year into account.

Once the training periods have been identified, there are specific training phases that need to be constructed, which are contained within the macro cycles. These training phases include the preparation period, which is normally split into the general preparation period (GPP) and the specific preparation period (SPP); the competition period (CP); and the transition recovery period (TRP). These training phases also contain the four core components that make up the season plan, i.e. technical, tactical, physical and psychological. Table 8.1 shows a basic example of a periodized plan for an English amateur soccer team, with four 12-week macro cycles, eight 6-week meso cycles and the specific training phases. Micro cycles have

85

Table 8.1 Basic periodized season plan for a soccer team

Macro 1			Macro 2			Macro 3			Macro 4		
Meso 1		Meso 2	Meso 3		Meso 4	Meso 5		Meso 6	Meso 7		Meso 8
Jul.	Aug.	Sep.	Oct.	Nov.	Dec.	Jan.	Feb.	Mar.	Apr.	May	Jun.
GPP		SPP	CP1			RP		CP2		TRP	

not been included in this example because of space restrictions, but an example of a full season plan for a university men's field hockey team, with the training periods, training phases, integration of the four core components, levels of intensity, testing and when to peak is shown in Appendix 9.

The focus of the GPP is general conditioning and is characterized by a large quantity of training at low intensities (Galvin and Ledger, 1998) and quite often performance in the competitive period has been determined by training achieved in this first period. The type of general conditioning that is conducted in the GPP depends much on the sport, but generally it should include a diet of aerobic and strength fitness training, some technical skills, and development of mental skills training. This may seem a lot to fit into a pre-season period, but the coach should be able to fully integrate the core components effectively.

The SPP is concerned with the introduction and development of the specific skills and technical patterns of the sport or event, and serves as a transition from general training to the competition period (Grosso, 2006). If the example of the English amateur soccer team is used again, pre-season friendly fixtures would feature in the SPP, technical skills and tactical concepts would be developed and reinforced, and mental skills training would be fully integrated into the training programme, such as pre-competition routines and goal setting. The SPP is shorter than the GPP and it may only take two to three weeks to progress from training to competition intensity (Galvin and Ledger, 1998). The CP is the period where training volume will decrease, but training intensity will either be maintained or increased. During this period competition situations are simulated, and training stress should be loaded to improve athletes' fitness levels, yet light enough to maintain motivation and energy levels (SOACG, 2007).

Although Galvin and Ledger propose that psychological and tactical preparation will take the place of physical and technical preparation during this period, this author would suggest that if players are able to train more than twice a week, there is still room to continue to reinforce technical skills throughout the season.

The final training phase is the TRP, and is concerned with recovery and having a break from training. This is not to suggest that the performer does no form of training. The performer(s) should do some form of general exercise to maintain a base level of physical fitness for an extended period and during the post-season. However, if the performer has gone through a period of intense competition, e.g. a tournament weekend followed by a midweek competition, then the coach should ensure that their performers have at least two or three days full rest to recuperate.

Periodization theory provides "a model for structuring athletes' training to achieve optimal performance, and many different interpretations of how to structure a periodized training programme have been proposed" (Cook, 2007, p. 10). However, it is up to the coach to decide on how they interpret the different models and perspectives and how they construct their season plan or training programme, because the demands of the sport and the structuring of a periodized plan should be tailored to the sport and individual.

Specifically, the coach has to decide on how long each training period and each training phase is, and in how much detail the four core components are implemented and delivered. However, the coach should consider utilizing season plan methodology in terms of having a framework with which to work. Ideally though, season plans should be individualized, because the individual performer is going to have different levels of fitness, technical ability, tactical understanding and psychological strength compared to his or her colleagues.

INDIVIDUALIZATION

The core principle of individualization is that coaches must "treat each athlete individually according to their abilities, potential, learning characteristics, and specifics of the sport, regardless of performance level" (Bompa, 1994, p. 37). Lyle (1996), cited in Cross and Lyle (2002, p. 174), suggests that "individualization is an essential element of the coaching process and has been identified as a key concept". Individualization is a complex process and the coach needs to consider a wide range of impacting factors when constructing an individualized training programme. For example, the coach would have to account for individual athletes' fitness and recovery rate; age; ability; gender; experience; motivation to train; time available to train; lifestyle factors, e.g. family, friends, finances; and work and education, all of which impact upon the coach when structuring the training load of the performer(s).

Table 8.2 shows an individualized training needs analysis, which the coach could use to identify individual factors that may enable him or her to construct an individualized training programme for his or her field hockey players. Although field hockey is used as an example, the criteria in the first column can be applied to any sport, and the coach's knowledge, coupled with discussion with the performer, can identify facilitating or limiting factors in constructing an individualized training programme.

With these areas identified, the coach can now construct an individualized training programme for each performer. If a defender is taken as an example, he is only able to train twice per week so his training load would have to be constructed accordingly, and the fact that he has a young family also impacts upon the amount of time he can train. Although he is reasonably well trained, there is an issue with his aerobic endurance therefore the coach may well incorporate some endurance training into the first of his weekly training sessions, such as interval training. The coach can link interval training in with a skills exercise, such as passing, by extending the amount of time the defender spends running in the exercise and shortening the recovery time, still with the focus on developing the skill of passing.

The second training session in the week could be utilized to account for the identified issues of defence awareness and concentration. The coach could plan a session working on the role of the defence and provide the defender with a mental skills package to improve his concentration. The skill for the coach is to identify all players' individual needs and see if a cluster of needs appears within one particular component. For example, if a cluster appears whereby three defenders and one midfielder require technical reinforcement of passing and first touch, and their aerobic fitness also requires attention, then a practice can be set up to account for these. This may seem a complicated and time consuming process for the team coach, and Cross and Ellis (1999) highlight that accounting for individualization in team sports can be a problem. Lyle (1992) and Cross and Lyle (1996), both cited in Cross and Lyle (2002), further suggest that time is a major factor for coaches in constructing an individualized training programme. However, this should not deter the coach from going through the process. The coach cannot operate with a "blanket approach" to their performers and individualization should be a process by which to account for all performers' individual needs.

Table 8.2 *Individualized training needs analysis*

Criteria	Performer 1 Defender	Performer 2 Midfielder	Performer 3 Forward
Age	30	20	22
Ability	Club	County	Regional
Gender	Male	Male	Male
Experience	18 years	8 years	10 years
Motivation	High	Low	High
Training time availability	Twice per week	Once per week	Three times per week
Impacting lifestyle factors	Has a young family	Works shifts in a local store	Financial – student
Fitness	Reasonably well trained; needs work on aerobic endurance; has trouble lasting a full game, and requires substituting	Muscular strength requires work, especially upper body; gets knocked off the ball easily	Requires work on explosive power; slow accelerating over the first five metres, which causes problems when trying to eliminate defenders
Technical	Passing out of defence	1st touch and vision	Foot work to get into a good goal scoring position
Tactical	Defence awareness	Link with defence and midfield	Lead runs and creation of personal space
Psychological	Concentration	Motivation and goal setting	Confidence

A good example of individualization being implemented at the elite level is provided by the Great Britain Hockey high performance coaching team in conjunction with an English Institute of Sport strength and conditioning coach. Prior to and after qualifying for the 2008 Beijing Olympics, the GB women were provided with individualized training programmes by an EIS strength and conditioning coach, plus appropriate work-life balance factors were also considered. GB Hockey negotiated with respective employers and universities for time for the GB women to allocate to training, and with this knowledge worked with the strength and conditioning coach to periodize the women's training programmes on an individual basis (Kerry, 2008).

PEAKING AND TAPERING

Peaking and tapering is another complex process within the complexities of planning, periodization and individualization. However, it is one of the coach's responsibilities to ensure that their performers reach peak performance, and therefore the coach must construct a programme that leads to optimal performance when it matters most (Bompa, 1994). Peaking is a process that in part is governed by adaptation to training effects, whereby the performer reaches optimal performance, and that has been facilitated by a well-designed, structured and effective training programme (Galvin and Ledger, 1998).

In working to lead performers to optimal performance the coach will have to consider when they want their performers to peak and how many times they want them to peak during a season or training programme. This will depend on when the important competition periods are, the relative importance of different competitions within the competition period, how many competitions there are and other factors suggested by Bompa (1994) that facilitate peaking, such as the performers' motivation, arousal, mental and physical recovery rate, technical and tactical ability and ability to adapt to different training loads. The stresses of training lead to adaptation, but also cause tiredness, which can inhibit a performer from reaching peak performance (Galvin and Ledger, 1998), and the coach should taper training in order for his or her performer to reach peak performance. Tapering training requires a reduction in training volume while increasing the intensity the performers train at, to simulate the competitive environment. Some coaches find this concept hard to grasp, as they believe that if they taper (reduce training volume) for more than just a few days, their performers' fitness and performance will suffer (Plowman and Smith, 2007). However, Costill, et al. (1985), along with many other researchers, have found that if intensity is maintained while training volume is reduced, physiological adaptations are retained and performance is either equalled or improved after a tapering of 7–21 days. The coach must be aware that when a tapering period follows a period of high training volume, the athlete may also feel uncoordinated and inefficient (Galvin and Ledger, 1998).

The challenge for the coach is to structure training so that peak performance can occur between the removal of fatigue and the reversal of training effects (Pankhurst, 2007). This challenge becomes further compounded for the team coach who has a number of players who all need to achieve peak performance at the same time.

SUMMARY

As well as short- and medium-term planning, the coach should also be able to construct long-term training programmes or season plans. Whether the coach is working in the high performance environment or at club level, there are a number of reasons why a season plan should be developed and implemented, such as establishing where your performer(s) are right now in terms of their technical ability, tactical knowledge, fitness and psychological needs; identifying where the performer(s), team or squad want to go; and provision of a programme that gives the coach and performer(s) a time-scale for the achievement of the identified goals.

A SWOT analysis can be a useful tool for the coach to identify strengths and weaknesses of their performers or opponents, which can inform construction of the season plan. On deciding on the length of the programme, the coach needs to think about the time-frames involved and how much time and how often the performers can spend on training. Once this has been established, a performance requirement analysis of the four core components (technical, tactical, physical and psychological) that make up the demands of the sport can be carried out so that they can be integrated into the overall training programme.

Once the coach has identified, collected and collated all the required information to put into the season plan, the next stage of the process is to divide the programme up into distinct training periods, and account for the process of periodization. The distinct training periods are called macro, meso and micro cycles. A macro cycle can be a prolonged period of time, and can be anything from a few months to several months; a meso cycle is a sub-cycle of the macro cycle, and the suggested duration is two–six weeks; the micro cycle is a sub-cycle of the meso cycle and is a training period of two–ten days, with training units (individual practice sessions) are incorporated into the micro cycles. Once the training periods have been identified, there are specific training phases that are required to be constructed, which include the preparation period, normally split into the general preparation period (GPP) and the specific preparation period (SPP), the competition period (CP) and the transition recovery period (TRP). These training phases also contain the four core components that make up the season plan – the technical, tactical, physical and psychological. Ideally, season plans should be individualized, because each performer is going have different levels of fitness, technical ability, tactical understanding and psychological strength in comparison to their colleagues. The core principle of individualization is one that coaches must "treat each athlete individually according to their abilities, potential, learning characteristics, and specifics of the sport, regardless of performance level" (Bompa, 1994, p. 37). Lyle (1996), cited in Cross and Lyle (2002, p. 174), suggests that "individualization is an essential element of the coaching process and has been identified as a key concept".

Peaking and tapering is another complex process within the complexities of planning, periodization and individualization. In working to lead performers to optimal performance, the coach will have considered when they want their performers to peak and how many times they want them to peak during a season or training programme. The stresses of training lead to adaptation, but also cause tiredness, which can inhibit a performer from reaching peak performance and the coach should taper training in order for the performer to reach peak performance. Tapering training means a reduction in training volume, which some coaches find hard to grasp, as they believe that if they taper (reduce training volume) for more than just a few days, their performers' fitness and performance will suffer (Plowman and Smith, 2007).

SEMINAR OR DISCUSSION QUESTIONS

1. Identify and describe the specific training phases in a season plan.
2. Explain the differences between peaking and tapering, and the relationship between training volume and training intensity.

KEY TERMS AND DEFINITIONS

- Competition period (CP) – the period where the objective is to compete consistently.
- General preparatory period (GPP) – general conditioning which is characterized by large quantities at low volume.
- Individualization – an individualized training programme.
- Macro cycle – long-term cycle.
- Meso cycle – medium-term cycle.
- Micro cycle – short-term cycle.
- Peaking – a process by which the performer reaches optimal physical performance.
- Periodization – division of a programme up into distinct training periods.
- Season plan – long-term scheme of work covering either an annual, biennial or quadrennial cycle.
- Specific preparatory period (SPP) – period for specific skill and technical development prior to the start of the competition period.

- SWOT analysis – process to identify Strengths, Weaknesses, Opportunities or Threats.
- Tapering – a reduction in training volume and an increase in training intensity.
- Training periods – macro, meso and micro cycles.
- Training unit – practice session.
- Transition recovery period (TPP) – recovery and having a break from training.

WEB LINKS

Training programmes – www.brianmac.co.uk
Training programmes – www.camelbackcoaching.com/training-programs.html

FURTHER READING

Bompa, T. (1994). *Periodization: Theory and Methodology of Training.* Human Kinetics, Champaign, IL.

Cook, M. (2007). Periodization theory: A refresher. *Coaching Edge,* 7, 10–11.

Cross, N. and Ellis, G. (2008). Performance Coaching: The individualization of training programmes. Online: http://www.coachesinfo.com/index.php?option=com_content&view=article&id=304:performance-coaching&catid=91:general-articles&Itemid=170 (accessed 14th October 2009).

Cross, N. and Lyle, J. (2002). *The Coaching Process: Principles and Practice for Sport.* Butterworth-Heinneman, Oxford.

Galvin, B. and Ledger, P. (1998). *A Guide to Planning Coaching Programmes.* Coachwise/SportsCoachUK, Leeds.

Grosso, M. R. (2006). Training theory: A primer on periodization. *The Coach,* 33, 25–33.

Pankhurst, A. (2007). *Planning and Periodization.* Coachwise/SportsCoachUK, Leeds, England.

Chapter 9

Management and the coach

⚡

CHAPTER OBJECTIVES

- Outline basic management theory.
- Describe human resource management.
- Identify and describe the role of the coach as a manager.
- Identify strategies the coach can use to maintain group control.
- Identify situations in which conflict may arise and explain how it can be resolved.

BASIC MANAGEMENT THEORY

Along with the many other roles that the coach fulfils, management and organization are key aspects of being an effective coach. Before management and organizational functions can be identified and applied to the coaching context, a basic understanding of the theoretical principles that underpin management practice is essential. Modern management principles emerged in the twentieth century, with different perspectives being offered to underpin and explain the management processes. Theories such as classical management emerged along with bureaucratic, scientific and administrative management perspectives, all of which focused on organizational efficiency (Barnett, 2009) and these persisted into the early 1900s (Torkildsen, 2005).

The human relations theory movement followed the classical management theory movement. This applied a more humanistic explanation to management theory which in practice suggested the focus should be on the individual. Human relations theory proposes that a motivated work force would be a more productive work force, thus benefitting the organization (McNamara, 2008).

The behaviourist movement of management theory received much attention during the 1950s and 1960s and evolved from classical management theory. The classical view of management theory was viewed by the behaviourist movement as a rather rigid perspective, and the behaviourists argued that "organization structures should be tempered with flexibility and a greater concern for employee involvement" (Torkildsen, 2005, p. 375).

In the 1960s Douglas McGregor, an American social psychologist, examined theories on how individuals behave at work and how best they can be managed and proposed a revolutionary perspective on management theory. McGregor argued for a Theory X and Theory Y model of management, whereby Theory X assumes that the average human being has an inherent dislike of work and will avoid it if they can, and Theory Y assumes staff act on their own initiative and invest effort in their work (Kopelman *et al.*, 2008). It was also suggested that Theory X managers will tend to push people to achieve a task, and Theory Y managers will tend to lead people to achieve a task (Torkildsen, 2005). Since the Theory X and Theory Y model, other management theoretical models have been proposed. They include: quantitative management theory, which deals in mathematical and statistical modelling and their use in decision making; systems theory, which views the organization as a group of interconnected parts with a common goal; and contingency theory, which has its foundations in the systems theory perspective but differs in that it recognizes and responds to different situations (Kriel, 2005).

Recently a culture has emerged in management organizations that emphasizes a client or customer focused approach, and a strong move has been made towards the empowerment of the individual in organizations. An approach that has gained significant momentum and support in recent years is total quality management (TQM). TQM is an approach to improving the effectiveness of an organization as a whole from top to bottom and bottom to top, and involves all employees in the process. Torkildsen (2005) and Zbaracki (1998) suggest that TQM is a better way to manage. TQM has spawned significant interest in management circles in the USA, and a number of organizations have adopted this management technique (Barron and Gjerde, 1996).

There are many other management theories that serve to explain the principles and practice of management and each has its own merits. Whatever management theoretical perspective the individual or organization comes from, an effective manager should exhibit good leadership skills, understand people, have wide a knowledge and experience of the organization and the role that he or she is in, display a degree of common sense and make good judgements (Torkildsen, 2005).

HUMAN RESOURCE MANAGEMENT

As well as having a good grounding in management theory the coach should also have a basic understanding of human resource management. Regardless of whether the coach is working at club level with just one assistant coach and parents as helpers, or in a High Performance Unit (HPU) with a team of coaches and specialists, the group or groups the coach works with are resources, and they need to be managed effectively. Human resource management is a "strategic and coherent approach to the management of the organization's most valued assets, principally the people who actually work for and contribute to the achievements of it objectives" (Armstrong, 2006, p. 3). Dawson (1993) suggests that the human resource manager is required to have certain levels of responsibility which may include human resource planning; industrial relations; welfare; recruitment and selection; training, development and induction; job evaluation; and performance appraisal. In order for the student to fully understand these responsibilities, they will now be applied in the coaching context, from the perspective of the coach being in a senior position at a club or in an organization.

The senior coach in their human resource planning role ensures that they have the correct policies and procedures in place to further recruit more coaches to support organizational needs. This may be a requirement at club level where more coaches are to be employed and deployed to support the junior section, or to support growth in the numbers of players at the club who require coaching. A further example of this would be a GBoS ensuring that enough coach educators are available to meet the demand of individuals wanting to attend coaching courses. Now that the coaching industry is increasingly falling under the umbrella of employment law, the senior coach of a club or organization should familiarize themselves with issues concerning industrial relations, which might include employment law, anti-discriminatory practice and contractual issues. The welfare of employees is also a responsibility of a manager, and in the coaching context the senior coach should have the welfare of his or her assistant coaches at heart, involving them in the decision-making process of developing, reflecting upon and evaluating session plans, and addressing any concerns that the assistant or junior coaches might have.

Recruitment and selection is another key responsibility of the senior coach, since they could be in a position at a club or large organization that needs to select and recruit a number of coaches. The senior coach together with a selection panel may interview potential coaches, ensuring that those coaches are suitable for the positions that have been advertised. Sport clubs who have a large player membership base can have a Director of Coaching that oversees coaching and the structure of coaching at the club. The Director of Coaching is usually a senior coach and will have the added responsibility of training and developing junior coaches, and any other coach who wishes to progress at the club. Coupled with this responsibility is job evaluation, where the senior coach will evaluate roles and responsibilities of the coaches at the club in order to ensure fairness in the distribution of coaching roles and responsibilities.

Finally, performance appraisal is a human resource management responsibility which should operate at all levels of coaching, regardless of whether the coach is in a senior position or not, and the coach should regularly provide feedback to their group of coaches or staff. This process could take place at the end of a coaching session with the senior coach providing positive feedback to an assistant coach who has just delivered a session, or appraising the performance of a group of coaches over a season.

When managing people the coach will need to consider the style in which they are managing. The same principles that are evident in coaching styles can be applied in the management of people, and different styles are required in a range of different situations. Nesti (1992) suggests that the management approach is different for organizations using volunteer staff and those employing paid staff. Specifically, a more autocratic management approach may be more effective for the paid employee (although this may not be viewed as attractive by the employee) and a more democratic management approach may be more effective for volunteer staff. Placing this in the coaching context, the paid staff, for example, could be the coaches and support staff working in the HPU, with the head coach being the senior manager delegating work and responsibilities, which may need a more autocratic leadership approach. The volunteer staff could be working in the club environment where the assistant coach might be a recently qualified coach, and the team of helpers are parents, which would require a more democratic, shared decision-making approach. Both these examples require a different style of management in order to get the best out of the staff (coaches) and more importantly for them to feel valued and that they all have a role to play.

THE COACH AS A MANAGER

By highlighting management theory and human resource management concepts and applications, the student should now have a basic understanding of the processes involved and how they can be applied in the coaching context. This section will take the coach as a manager a stage further by identifying specific management tasks and responsibilities that may be required of the coach. This is not to say that the coach should be over-burdened with all the management roles and responsibilities; they should be in a position to delegate to others, such as the captain or other members of a team. For example, in many UK universities the coach is just responsible for the delivery of practices. The captain takes responsibility for selection and team affairs on the pitch and the team members take divided responsibility for the team finances, social activities, sourcing of kit and standing as the club chairman. In the USA the collegiate system is different, whereby a structured athletic programme negates the need for the players to take on responsibilities other than just playing, and the coach takes on a multitude of other roles.

Time management is one of the fundamental aspects of management, and the coach should set a good example by arriving at practices, venues and meetings in plenty of time. The more efficiently the coach manages their performers the more time they will have to coach them (Martens, 2004). Poor time management not only affects planning and delivery of elements in the coaching process, it can also have an impact upon players, assistant coaches and support staff. Kozoll (1988) suggests that good time management can mean the difference between an effective and an ineffective training programme or practice session. It is not good coaching practice to turn up late, as this sends out the wrong message to the athlete, and leaves the coach with reduced time to do whatever they have to do.

Chambers (1997) suggests that the coach has many roles to perform, and that there are management and administrative tasks that are common to all sports, which are divided into three categories: pre-, during and post-season management. However, Martens (2004) is more detailed in identifying seven different management roles that the coach needs to master or at least delegate the responsibilities of to an assistant coach. These are the policy, information, personnel, instructional, competition, logistic and, financial and event and contest management roles. The coach may be required to develop and implement policies such as team selection, attendance at training or a disciplinary policy in the day-to-day running of a team or squad of players in order to maintain a level of structure and set boundaries. Collecting and collating information such as records of fitness tests is an administrative task that requires a sensitive management approach in terms of ensuring that any confidential information is stored safely.

One of the understated management tasks that the coach has to contend with is accounting for players' and support staff's needs and aspirations and their activities in and out of the competitive arena, rewarding and appraising individuals when appropriate. The coach also has to manage the immediate practice environment and by taking an instructional approach set goals, construct session and season plans and evaluate the performers and themselves, as well as the programme's effectiveness. The coach may also be involved in planning and organizing competitions and tournaments, which requires a good understanding of tournament rules and regulations. In some instances the coach may also be responsible for transportation, equipment, hiring of facilities, health and safety issues, and risk assessments, which would fall under the guise of logistical management.

Finally, the coach may also have financial responsibilities, which might include collection of match fees, subscriptions, obtaining funds through sponsorship, preparing budgets and balancing income over expenditure during a season. Martens (2004) provides a comprehensive list of different management categories that are appropriate in the North American culture of sports coaching and the collegiate system. However, in the UK the organization of sports clubs in comparison to the North American system is somewhat different. For example, the coach working at club level in many sports will rarely have responsibility for the finances – that onus usually falls on the club treasurer or the captain at the team level, in terms of collecting match fees.

Event, contest and league management is organized primarily by the GBoS, and at the regional level for local leagues and competitions. Generally, responsibility for facilities and match fixtures is delegated to someone nominated at the club or organization. Transportation at the amateur level is usually organized by the team, who decide who is driving to the venue and how many cars are needed, but if the coach is working with a manager or assistant coach then this may be delegated to them.

In reality, and especially when considering the amateur aspect of sport in the UK, only four (policy, information, personnel and instruction management) from the seven categories are applicable. In professional sport in the UK these categories may even be limited to the coach being just an instructional manager, with other individuals in the organization being paid to fulfil the remaining six roles.

MANAGING THE COACHING ENVIRONMENT – MAINTAINING GROUP CONTROL

When considering a "belts and braces" approach to coaching practice, another management skill which the coach should develop is being able to maintain control of his or her group when delivering a practice. This should not be perceived as an authoritarian issue but one of organizational management, in terms of gaining and maintaining the attention of your players and ensuring that instructions are understood. To effectively organize the group the coach may have to carry out the following:

- Plan the practice session.
- Start and finish the session on time.
- Maintain an appropriate level of discipline and a safe environment.
- Provide unambiguous verbal instructions.
- Check players' understanding of the instructions.
- Vary the activities.
- Limit distractions and keep players focused.
- Challenge inappropriate behaviour – abide by the Code of Conduct for Sports Coaches.
- Intervene in sessions only when appropriate.

(Robinson, 2006b)

CONFLICT RESOLUTION

The reality is that conflict is unavoidable for even the most careful and passive person, and unfortunately conflict permeates all areas of our lives. Because emotions can run high in many sporting situations, the coach can often find themselves having to resolve conflict. Most teams will occasionally encounter some conflict, which is not a huge problem, but constant and protracted conflict can affect the cohesion of a team, and is energy inefficient – the energy could be best spent in performance (Thomas, 2000). Miscommunication (verbal or non-verbal) is arguably one of the main sources of conflict, and can occur if the coach does not communicate the right information, communicates negatively, does not give all the information to the performer or the performer who receives the information misinterprets the message.

Another source of conflict is the coach setting ineffective goals for the individual or group, which they may feel are not attainable or challenging enough. Ineffective or unacceptable methods of coaching are a further source of conflict, e.g. the performer(s) may not like the coach's autocratic coaching style, or the way practices are structured. Constant criticism,

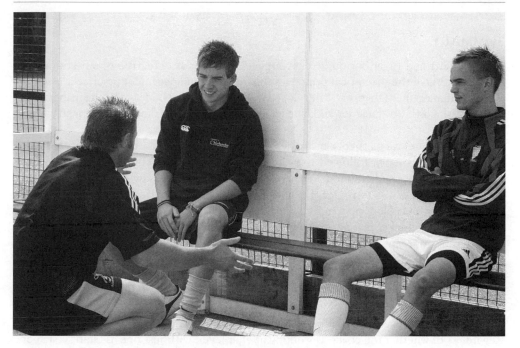

Photo 9.1 A coach resolving conflict between two performers.

berating of players, confrontational behaviour and a general negative attitude can be further sources of conflict between coach and performer which ideally should be avoided. However, conflict does not just arise between the coach and performers; it can also arise between players, between players and officials, and between players, parents, observers and spectators.

Thomas (2000) suggests that four types of conflict exist: within the individual player, within the team, between team members and between coach and team. The individual player can experience lack of confidence in their ability or performance, which can manifest as self-induced conflict about not being selected for the team. Conflict within a team can increase team anxiety, inhibit skill learning, undermine the authority of the coach and can contribute to coaching burnout (Martinek, 1991). Conflict between team members can be due to a range of issues, from just not liking someone in the team, personal issues being bought into the sporting environment, disagreements in team selection or rivalry. What is certain, however, is that the smallest issue can be magnified in the team setting and affect the productivity and cohesion of the group. Conflict between the coach and team can manifest in various ways, from the coach not sharing views, concerns and information with the players, not clarifying roles and responsibilities, not clarifying tactics or generally performing poorly (Thomas, 2000).

Conflict should be handled in a constructive way, otherwise the relationship between the parties involved could break down, and their behaviour could become further entrenched. There are general strategies that the coach can use to handle or resolve conflict, such as trying intervene as soon as possible; defusing the situation; trying not to be judgemental until the full facts of the conflict are known; mediating if possible; encouraging those involved to resolve any differences and managing the situation to avoid further potential conflict (Robinson, 2006b).

SUMMARY

Management and organization are key aspects of being an effective coach and a basic understanding of the theoretical principles that underpin management practice is essential. Classical management theory was developed in order to try and understand the management process. It focused on efficiency and bureaucratic, scientific and administrative management processes.

The human relations theory movement, seeking to provide a more human approach to management theory, followed the classical management theory movement and was itself followed by the behaviourist theory movement, which saw the classical view of management theory as too rigid. Douglas McGregor, an American social psychologist, proposed a revolutionary perspective on management theory and argued for a Theory X and Theory Y model of management, whereby Theory X assumed that the average human being has an inherent dislike of work and will avoid it if they can, and Theory Y assumed that staff act on their own initiative and invest effort in their work (Torkildsen, 2005). Recently a culture has emerged in management organizations that emphasizes a client- or customer-focused approach, and a strong move has been made towards the empowerment of the individual in organizations.

The TQM perspective is the prevailing contemporary notion of management theory. Regardless of whether the coach is working at club level, with just one assistant coach and parents as helpers, or in a HPU with a team of coaches and specialists, the group or groups the coach works with are resources, and they need to be managed effectively. Dawson (1993) suggests that the human resource manager is required to have certain levels of responsibility which may include human resource planning; industrial relations; welfare; recruitment and selection; training, development and induction; job evaluation; and performance appraisal. As the coach progresses and attains higher coaching qualifications they will find that they are more involved in human resource management and the development of other coaches than when they were just starting out in their career. This therefore requires that the coach has knowledge of management principles, and a skill set in order to manage effectively.

Chambers (1997) argues that the coach has many roles to perform, and that there are administrative tasks that are common to all sports, which are divided into three categories: pre-, during and post-season management. However, Martens (2004) identifies seven different management role categories that the coach might be required to fulfil. There are the policy, personnel, instructional, logistics, information, financial and event and contest management roles. Taking a very basic approach, the coach has to manage the coaching environment during the practice session in terms of gaining and maintaining the attention of players and ensuring that instructions are understood.

Unfortunately, the coach will have to deal with and resolve conflict at some stage in their career, and choices have to be made regarding selection and tactics, which at times are not going to be popular. Conflict management and resolution is therefore a skill that the coach should try to develop.

SEMINAR OR DISCUSSION QUESTIONS

1. Identify and describe Dawson's (1993) seven levels of human resource management responsibility and apply them to a coaching context.
2. Identify the sources of conflict that may arise between a coach and his or her performers and identify strategies to resolve issues.

KEY TERMS AND DEFINITIONS

- Behavioural management theory – a flexible and employee-involved approach.
- Classical management theory – focuses on efficiency and includes bureaucratic, scientific and administrative management.
- Conflict resolution – intervention by a coach or other person to manage disagreements between individuals.
- Contingency theory – when applying management, different situations are recognized and responded to.
- Human relations management theory – provides a more human perspective on management theory.
- Human resource management – the effective management of people.
- Management theory – a principal idea that provides a framework with which to understand the processes that are involved in management.
- Managing the coaching environment – maintaining group control of a practice session.
- Quantitative management theory – deals in mathematical and statistical modelling and their use in decision making.
- Systems theory – views the organization as a group of interconnected parts with a common goal.

WEB LINKS

Institute of Leisure and Amenity Management (ILAM) – www.ispal.org.uk
Institute of Sport and Recreation Management (ISRM) – www.isrm.co.uk
Management history – www.managementhelp.org/mgmnt/history.htm

FURTHER READING

Chambers, D. (1997). *Coaching: The Art and the Science*. Key Porter, Toronto.
Kozoll, C. (1988). *Coaches' Guide to Time Management*. Springfield Books Ltd, England.
Martens, R. (2004). *Successful Coaching* (3rd edn). Human Kinetics, Champaign, IL.
Thomas, A. (2000). Managing conflict. *Faster, Higher, Stronger*, 9, 26–7.
Torkildsen, G. (2005). *Leisure and Recreation Management*. Routledge, London.
Watt, D. C. (2003). *Sports Management and Administration* (2nd edn). Routledge, London.

Part 4

Anatomy and physiology, training principles and the coach

INTRODUCTION

This part of the book provides a general yet comprehensive outline of the knowledge that the coach needs of anatomical and physiological structure and function, and the training principles that the coach will need to implement and integrate into their training programmes and practice sessions.

Chapter 10 outlines basic anatomical and physiological concepts, such as the terms that are associated with movement, the nature and function of the skeleton, types of bone and function of joints and muscles. An anterior and posterior diagram view of the skeleton is also provided so that the student can identify the location of major bones in the body. The nature and function of the heart, lungs and digestive system are also highlighted in Chapter 10, and are supported with diagrams that identify the location of the key areas of the organs. Aerobic and anaerobic functioning is examined in detail, and the energy systems such as the adenosine tri-phosphate, creatine, anaerobic glycolysis and aerobic systems that enable the body to perform maximally and effectively are highlighted. Nutrition and hydration also feature in Chapter 10, in terms of taking a fundamental look at nutritional intake for sport performance and how the performer should hydrate effectively in order to maintain homeostasis in body functioning.

Chapter 11 examines the fundamentals of training and fitness, specifically the role of the coach integrating and implementing fitness programmes. Chapter 11 also identifies and describes the principles and components of fitness and fitness training methods, such as interval and Fartlek training. Fitness testing and the types of test that the coach can utilize when assessing the performer's fitness are identified. The nature of strength and conditioning and the role of the strength and conditioning coach are also discussed in Chapter 11. A case study features a professional fitness trainer who implements fitness training programmes for sports teams in the UK.

Chapter 12 examines the concept of injury prevention and highlights warming up and cooling down principles, the concept of warm-up decrement and developments in injury prevention such as using ice baths. At the end of the chapter suggested seminar or discussion questions are provided, along with key terms and definitions. Web links and suggested further readings are also provided if more information or further research is required

Chapter 10

Anatomy and physiology

CHAPTER OBJECTIVES

- Identify and describe anatomical and physiological function.
- Identify and describe terms associated with body movement.
- Identify and describe the structure and function of the skeleton, muscles, heart, lungs and digestive system.
- Identify and describe the different energy systems.
- Explain how the performer should hydrate and fuel for performance.

ANATOMICAL AND PHYSIOLOGICAL FUNCTION

In order to prepare the performer physically and implement fitness and training programmes, the coach should have a sound knowledge of anatomy and physiology, and understand how the body works. The human body is made up of different systems such as the skeletal, muscular, circulatory, respiratory, nervous, hormonal, digestive and excretory systems. Although these systems are separate, they do not function in isolation of each other; they are linked in order to facilitate effective functioning of the body at rest and during exercise.

TERMS ASSOCIATED WITH BODY MOVEMENT

In sport the body is required to execute a range of movement in different directions to either run, swim, jump, catch, kick, throw or hit a ball with a stick, racket, club or bat. The coach requires a sound knowledge of the way these movements are described, and the function of specific anatomical parts that impact on the ability of the performer to execute a skill. These movements include:

- Flexion – the bending of a body part, so that the two parts are bought together, e.g. bringing the hand to the shoulder by bending at the elbow.
- Extension – the moving apart of two limbs, e.g. the straightening of the arm by bending the elbow, so the forearm moves away from the shoulder.
- Plantarflexion – moving and placing the foot down away from the shin using the ankle joint.
- Dorsiflexion – moving the foot towards the shin using the ankle joint.

- Abduction – moving of a body segment (limb) sideways, away from the body, e.g. moving the leg sideways and outwards at the hip.
- Adduction – moving a body segment towards the body.
- Lateral flexion – bending of the trunk to one side, either left or right.
- Medial rotation – rotation of a limb segment, e.g. turning the leg inwards so that the toes point inwards.
- Lateral rotation – rotation of a limb segment, e.g. turning the leg outwards so that the toes point outwards.
- Supination – movement of the forearm so that the palm faces upwards or forwards.
- Pronation – movement of the forearm so that the palm faces downwards.
- Inversion – turning the inside edge of the foot upwards.
- Eversion – turning the outside edge of the foot upwards.

(Adapted from Palastanga *et al.*, 1998)

STRUCTURE AND FUNCTION OF THE SKELETON

The skeleton is a framework that has many joint connections, providing physical support and shape for the body and at the same time protection for the internal organs. The skull protects the brain, the vertebral column the spinal cord and the rib cage protects the heart and lungs. The infant body contains 350 bones, but these fuse together over time, so that the adult body contains 250 bones, over half of which are in the hands and feet (Hardman and Stensel, 2003). Throughout childhood and into adulthood cartilage changes into bone through a process called ossification; calcium is laid down in the bones making them hard and collagen fibres are produced which make the bones light (Beashel and Taylor, 1997). Red and white blood cells and a range of minerals essential for growth and repair are also produced in the bone marrow of the skeleton (Davis *et al.*, 1995). There are four main types of bone which are classified by shape:

1. The *long* bones are located in the arms and legs, and are used for major body movements.
2. The *short* bones can be found in the hands and feet, and are used for fine movement.
3. The *flat* bones include cranial bones (the skull), the sternum (breastbone), the ribs and scapula (the shoulder blade); they protect vital organs.
4. *Irregular* bones include the vertebral column, and bones in the face.

(Adapted from Bartlett, 1997)

A further two types of bones are classified by their location. The sutural bones are located between the joints of certain cranial bones and vary between individuals, and the sesamoid bones, which are load-bearing bones, can also exhibit individual differences, e.g. the patella (the knee cap bone) (Bartlett, 1997). The skeleton is divided into the axial and appendicular skeletons. The axial skeleton consists of the skull, vertebral column, ribs and sternum, and the appendicular skeleton consists of the arms and legs, shoulders and hip girdle. The spinal column is made up of 33 small bones called vertebrae, and between each of these is a thin layer of cartilage called a vertebral disc, which acts as a shock absorber. The vertebral column supports the upper body and protects the spinal cord (Beashel and Taylor, 1997). Figure 10.1 shows anterior and posterior views of the skeleton.

Bones of the skeleton are connected by joints and a range of different joint types exists in the human body, each of which has a different function. The joints are categorized into three

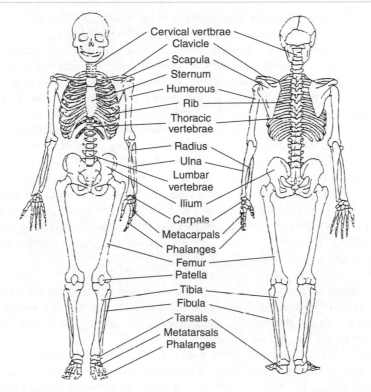

Figure 10.1 Anterior and posterior view of skeleton.
Source: Bartlett (1997, Figure 1.9, p. 16).

types: immovable joints, which are found between the flat bones of the skull; slightly movable joints, which are found in the joints of the vertebral column and the ribs and sternum; and freely movable joints, which are also known as synovial joints and are found in many parts of the body, including the hip, elbow and ankle (Bartlett, 1997). The synovial joints are lubricated with synovial fluid, which allows for free movement of the joint. Ligaments are attached to joints and their function is to hold the bones together at the joint, limit the range of movement and prevent dislocation (Beashel and Taylor, 1997; Bartlett, 1997; Davis *et al.*, 1995). A common sports injury is the tearing or rupturing of ligaments, which is usually due to the over-extension of a range of movement that the joint was designed for.

There are six basic types of synovial joint: the ball and socket joint, which moves freely in all directions (found for example in the hip and shoulder); the pivot joint for which rotation is only possible (located between the first and second cervical vertebrae in the neck); the hinge joint, which moves one way only (found for example in the elbow); the gliding joint (found for example in the carpal bones in the hand); the saddle joint (found for example in the thumb) and the condyloid joint (found for example in the knuckle) (Bartlett, 1997; Wirhead, 1984).

STRUCTURE AND FUNCTION OF MUSCLES

Identifying and understanding the functions of different muscles and their location is fundamental for the coach. The coach should know the roles of different muscles that determine execution of a skill, and the sequence of movement of different muscle groups – otherwise there will be the potential for injury and ineffective skill execution. Movement occurs in sport because muscles shorten (contract) and lengthen (extend) to either run, jump, catch, kick or throw and there are over 600 voluntary muscles in the body (Beashel and Taylor, 1997). This constant movement of contraction and extension generates body heat, gives us our own individual shape, protects our abdominal organs and circulates the blood (Hay and Reid, 1988).

There are three different types of muscle: striated (skeletal), smooth and cardiac. Striated muscles are attached to the skeleton and are controlled consciously when the person decides to move, and are often called voluntary muscles (McLaughlin *et al.*, 2006). Cardiac muscle is myogenic, which means it contracts automatically without requiring nervous stimulation (Clegg, 1995). Smooth muscles are mostly found in layers; they form the muscle part of the digestive tract, the bladder, blood vessels and the skin, and are often called involuntary muscles. Every movement involves a group of muscles working together and each has a specific role (McLaughlin *et al.*, 2006). This is known as the group of action muscles, and the individual roles are as follows:

- Agonist (prime mover) – this is the muscle primarily responsible for a given movement, e.g. the agonist for the sit-up is the rectus abdominus (main stomach muscle).
- Antagonist – this is the muscle that relaxes as the prime mover contracts, e.g. the antagonist for the arm dip is the bicep.
- Synergist – there are two types of synergist. The helping synergist helps the prime mover, e.g. the helping synergists for the sit-up with rotation are the internal obliques and the rectus abdominus. The true synergist contracts to block any unwanted movement, e.g. if the prime mover has two actions and only one is required. When one is drinking, the prime mover is the biceps brachii, whose actions are flexion at the elbow and supination at the elbow, the brachioradialis prevents unwanted movement (supination of the elbow).
- Fixator – this is a muscle that contracts (usually isometrically) statically to hold a joint or body part stable during a movement and keep a joint in position while enabling the agonist to function. An example of this would be the elbow muscles keeping the elbow stable while a cricketer is bowling a delivery.

(Adapted from Clegg, 1995 and Rowett, 1999)

Muscle contractions are divided into three categories: isotonic, isometric and isokinetic. An isotonic contraction is one in which the muscle tension stays the same and the muscle length shortens; an isometric contraction is one in which muscle tension is generated and the muscle length stays the same; and an isokinetic contraction is one in which the muscle shortens at a constant speed and exerts maximum tension over the full range of movement (Clegg, 1995). When the muscle is shortened it is known as a concentric action and when the muscle is lengthened is it known as an eccentric action (Beashel and Taylor, 1997). A good proportion of eccentric muscle contractions involve lowering the body to the floor and are negative movements, working against gravity (Rowett,1999).

Figure 10.2a shows an anterior and figure 10.2b a posterior view of the major muscles in the body. Muscle is composed of actin molecules, which make up the actin (thin) filament, and myosin molecules which make up the myosin (thick) filament. Both filaments are encased by the myofibril (the contractile elements of the cell), hundreds of which are banded together so that they run the length of each cell (Rowett, 1999). The cell (muscle fibre) encases the myofibril, and extends from one bone to another. These muscle fibres then make up bundles

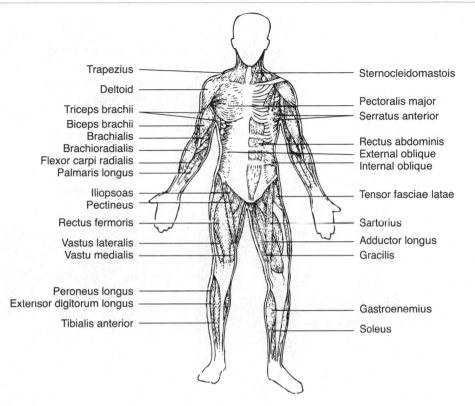

Figure 10.2a Anterior view of the major muscles in the body.

Source: Bartlett (1997, Figure 1.15a, p. 30).

of fibres that form the skeletal muscle (Tortora and Grabowski, 1996). There are two different muscle fibre types called slow twitch and fast twitch muscle fibres. The fast twitch fibres are further divided into fast twitch glycolytic and fast twitch oxidative fibres. The oxidative fibres have a better oxygen supply and are able to be optimized for aerobic activities. The human body has equal amounts of each fibre type, but there are individual differences (Quinn, 2007).

Generally, it is the endurance-type athletes, such as marathon runners and long distance swimmers, who have more slow twitch fibres, and the power athletes such as weightlifters, sprinters, javelin and shot put throwers who have more fast twitch fibres. Slow twitch fibres are slower contractors and are able to work for extended periods without tiring and take longer to contract. Fast twitch fibres contract very quickly, tire quickly and are used in explosive-type activities.

NATURE AND FUNCTION OF THE HEART

The heart is situated in the chest cavity underneath the sternum and between the lungs, slightly to the left of the centre of the body. It is roughly the size of a closed fist, and beats around 100,000 times per day, pumping around 7,600 litres of blood daily, or 70 millilitres per beat, and weighs between 250–350 grams (McKardle *et al.*, 2007). The heart is a dual-action pump in which both sides of the heart contract at the same time, although each side

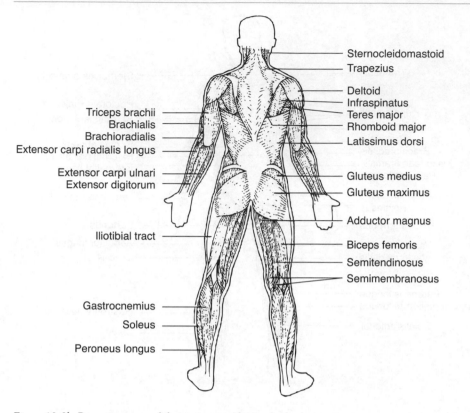

Figure 10.2b Posterior view of the major muscles in the body.
Source: Bartlett (1997, Figure 1.15b p. 31).

is functionally different. A network of blood vessels makes up the structure of the heart and the circulatory fluid that flows around and through the heart is blood. Deoxygenated blood circulates through the body via the venae cavae into the right atrium and then into the right ventricle and to the lungs via the pulmonary arteries. The lungs then return oxygenated blood via the pulmonary veins into the left atrium and then into the left ventricle and to the main aorta (Clegg, 1995). The main aorta then supplies oxygenated blood to the body, vital organs and the brain. Cardiac contractions enable the pumping of the blood through the heart and are initiated by electrical impulses which permeate through a network of fibres throughout the ventricular walls, causing the ventricles to contract and consequently the heart to pump (Davis *et al.*, 1995).

Figure 10.3 shows the structure of the heart. The heart consists of the following major parts: the pericardium or heart wall which is made up of myocardium muscle; four major chambers, two atria and two ventricles; the interventricular septum or dividing wall; valves that open and shut to allow blood flow. The heart's blood supply comes from the coronary artery, the pulmonary artery, the aorta and the superior and inferior venae.

NATURE AND FUNCTION OF THE LUNGS

Breathing is under neural control, which means breathing is controlled by involuntary, automatic nerve impulses from the central nervous system (brain) (McKardle *et al.*, 2007). The

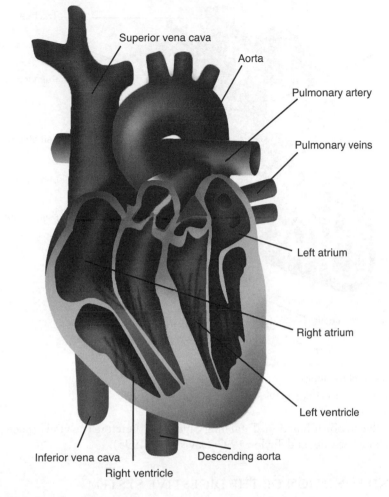

Superior vena cava

Aorta

Pulmonary artery

Pulmonary veins

Left atrium

Right atrium

Left ventricle

Inferior vena cava

Descending aorta

Right ventricle

Figure 10.3 Structure of the heart.

Source: Adapted from Beashel and Taylor (1997).

respiratory system has two major functions: pulmonary ventilation and external respiration (Palastanga *et al.*, 1998). The process of inspiration and expiration to fill and empty the lungs is facilitated by the contraction and relaxation of the external intercostal muscles in the rib cage. In broad terms, the respiratory system consists of a windpipe which divides into two bronchial tubes. These branch out into bronchioles which then expand into small clusters of air cells called the alveoli. The alveolar walls consist of a single layer and have a large surface area. A small network of blood capillaries in the walls of the alveoli provides a surface for the actual process of gaseous exchange. Gaseous exchange is the process of oxygen and carbon dioxide moving between the lungs and blood and involves the removal of carbon dioxide through a process of passive diffusion (Powers and Howley, 1997).

Figure 10.4 shows the structure of the lungs. Resting air moves in and out of the lungs with each breath taken, and this is called the tidal volume. After each breath there is always some air left in the lungs, which is called the residual volume. The vital capacity is the largest amount of air that can be expelled out from the lungs after the individual has taken in as

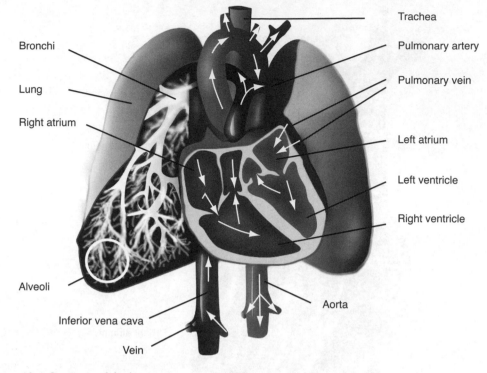

Figure 10.4 Structure of the lungs.

Source: Adapted from Beashel and Taylor (1997).

much air as possible in one inhalation. Total lung capacity is therefore the vital capacity plus the residual volume (Beashel and Taylor, 1997; Davis *et al.*, 1995).

NATURE AND FUNCTION OF THE DIGESTIVE SYSTEM

The digestive system breaks down the food we eat in order for it to pass through our bloodstream, releasing nutrients to promote cell and tissue growth for our day-to-day energy requirements (Vander *et al.*, 1998). The food is eaten and pushed down the gullet and into the stomach. In the stomach the food is mixed with gastric juices, enzymes and diluted acid which break down the food (Beashel and Taylor, 1997). The food then moves through the duodenum and into the small intestine. In the small intestine alkaline enzymes are added to the food, and it is further broken down and nutrients are transported into the blood. Any waste products pass into the large intestine, stay there for around 12 hours during which most of the water and remaining nutrients are removed (Beashel and Taylor, 1997). The solidified remains transit the large intestine and leave the body through the anus, and the fluid waste is passed as urine (McLaughlin *et al.*, 2006).

The digestive system requires blood flow and oxygen to facilitate the process of breaking down food and converting it into nutrients and energy. When exercising, blood flow to the digestive organs is reduced, as is oxygen because blood flow and oxygen are directed to the muscles for exercise. This competition for blood flow and oxygen inhibits the digestive process (Richfield, 2008). Taking this into account, the coach should ensure that their athletes do not eat a heavy meal for at least two hours before they train, otherwise their digestive systems will not receive the adequate blood flow to break down the food in the stomach. Quite often if the performer has eaten a heavy meal and then begins training they will feel sluggish and their muscles will feel heavy; this is possibly because less than sufficient blood flow is being directed towards the muscles for exercise (Richfield, 2008). A further reason not to eat a heavy meal before training or competition is that food can lie in the stomach waiting to be broken down. A full stomach can push up into the diaphragm, which may affect the effectiveness of breathing.

ENERGY SYSTEMS

The adenosine tri-phosphate and creatine phosphate systems

The immediate energy system utilized in the body for physical activity is the ATP (adenosine tri-phosphate) system. The supply of ATP only lasts for a few seconds, and there is a need to recoup ATP quickly, which is achieved by the breakdown of creatine phosphate (CrP) (Shepherd, 2006). Once this energy supply is depleted, the body has to draw on the lactic energy system, which requires the utilization of glycogen to provide more ATP (Tortora and Grabowski, 1996).

The anaerobic (lactic acid) system

The anaerobic system does not rely on oxygen and is utilized when the body is working at maximum effort and the fuel and oxygen requirements exceed the rate of supply to the muscles so that they have to draw on a reserve store of fuel. This system is utilized to great effect by sports that require explosive power, such as 100-metre sprinters. The anaerobic system supplies energy from around 20 seconds to around two minutes (Maughan and Gleeson, 2004). When the muscles run out of this source of fuel after a short period, the lack of oxygen in the muscles means they go into what is called oxygen debt and lactic acid builds up in the muscle. This point is called the lactate or anaerobic threshold, described as the "onset of blood lactate accumulation (OBLA), and is considered to be at around 65%–80% of VO_2 max in trained athletes and 50%–60% of VO_2 max in untrained athletes" (Powers and Howley, 1997, p. 51).

The coach should understand that when explosive-type activities which are anaerobically demanding are to be integrated into the training session, there will have to be recovery periods for the performers between practices. If the coach does not allow for recovery periods then the lactic acid which can build up in the muscles will not have the chance to dissipate through the normal processes; the performers will tire quickly; it will be noticeable that skills will break down very quickly; and the required sprint or jog back to a recovery position will become a walk. The body is adaptable and limited activity can resume after some of the oxygen debt has been repaid. However, it is impossible for the coach to measure an individual's oxygen debt during training; therefore the coach needs to understand there is a limit in anaerobic functioning and that there will be a gradual decrease in physical performance, which means the practice has to be structured accordingly.

The aerobic system

The aerobic system works when enough oxygen is being supplied to the muscles, and the body is working at a level that the demands for oxygen and fuel are met by the body's intake. When the muscles are provided with enough oxygen, carbohydrate is first broken down into energy, and once this store has been depleted the body's fat stores are utilized for energy. Earlier studies demonstrated that carbohydrate was the preferential fuel for endurance exercise, but more recent studies have suggested a greater role for fats than was previously thought (Hagerman, 1992).

For the endurance performer, such as marathon runners, Tour de France cyclists and tri-athletes, the aerobic system is important. For the coach, understanding the function and limitations of the aerobic system is equally as important, because educating and advising the performer on training intensity and volume, and the types of training that will make effective improvements in aerobic functioning and capacity can be a significant part of the coach's role. Furthermore, when the coach is assessing the demands of their sport in putting together a season plan, it may be that the pre-season phase requires a lot of work at low intensity but with high volume aerobic conditioning, therefore having a good understanding of the aerobic system will enable the coach to structure a training programme that is effective and that suits the needs of the individual performer.

In order to keep our muscles supplied with energy for extended periods of activity, the cardio-respiratory system (heart, lungs and blood vessels) needs to be developed; the term aerobic capacity refers to the cardio-respiratory system's ability to deal with extended bouts of physical activity. A performer's maximum aerobic capacity is commonly known as their VO_2 max, and is the maximum amount of oxygen that can be transported to and used by the muscles in an individual (Shepherd, 2006). The VO_2 max is the gold standard of cardio-respiratory fitness (Powers and Howley, 1997). Once the VO_2 max is determined, the performer's aerobic threshold is known and prolonged and continuous physical activity above this threshold will improve aerobic fitness. The performer's heart rate should be kept at around 70–85 per cent of his or her maximum heart rate in order to improve aerobic capacity (Beashel and Taylor, 1997).

The estimation of maximum heart rate has been a feature of exercise physiology and applied sciences since the 1930s, and has largely been based on the formula $HR_{max}= 220$ age (Robergs and Landwehr, 2002). This unfortunately has no scientific merit for use in exercise physiology and related fields. A new equation has emerged ($208 \div 0.7 \times$ age), suggested by Tanaka *et al.* (2001) to be more accurate in determining the estimation of maximum heart rate. Laboratory tests using a range of equipment and sports science expertise can be used to determine VO_2 max. However, if the coach is operating in isolation then field-based fitness tests can be used as a general predictor of aerobic capacity.

It is worth considering at this point that there is a gradual decrease in the uptake of each energy system. Each system does not just stop; there is a gradual decrease of one, then there is a gradual uptake of the next system and so forth, but even then there is a limit to the body's ability to continue prolonged bouts of physical activity without replenishing the energy systems and giving the body a chance to recover.

NUTRITION AND HYDRATION – FUELLING FOR PERFORMANCE

The body needs fuel in order to carry out day-to-day activities and although the UK Department of Health recommends that the average daily caloric intake for men should be 2,250 calories and women 1,940 calories (Geddes and Grossett, 1995), there are individual differences and certainly the sports performer will have varying requirements dependent on the sport and level of physical activity being carried out. Michael Phelps, the US record-breaking, eight-time gold medal winner at the 2008 Beijing Olympic Games, is reported to consume 12,000 calories a day to enable him to have enough energy fuel to train and compete

(Henley, 2008). A coach is in a good position to educate the performer in the basics of fuelling effectively for performance, however, any specialist dietary needs and supplementation information should be provided by a sports nutritionist. The sports performer should still have a balanced diet that consists of around 60 per cent of carbohydrate, 25 per cent fat and 15 per cent protein, but again this will vary depending on the type of training being carried out and the sport.

Carbohydrates are stored as glycogen in the liver and muscles and they are a quick and efficient source of energy (Maughan et al., 1997). Sports performers require a lot of carbohydrates as an energy source to provide fuel for the muscles, and carbohydrates are broken down into two types. Complex carbohydrates (starches) are naturally occurring in bread, rice, pasta and wheat (cereals, porridge). These are slow-release carbohydrates, which keep the individual fuller for longer and release energy to the body more efficiently and slowly. Simple carbohydrates (simple sugars) are found in processed food in which sugar is added, such as sweets, biscuits and cakes. Simple carbohydrates give a quick energy boost and are limited nutritionally. Simple carbohydrates are often found in processed foods, which can also contain hidden fats like trans fats. These trans fats are chemically altered vegetable oils and are found in thousands of processed foods and have been linked to high cholesterol (FSA, 2008), which can lead to heart attacks and strokes.

Fats are an important source of fuel and energy for the sports performer. Their energy release is much slower than carbohydrates' and more oxygen is required to break down fat compared to carbohydrates. Towards the end of prolonged exercise, when glycogen reserves become depleted, fat supplies can make up 80 per cent of the total energy requirement (McKardle et al., 2007). Once marathon runners have used up their carbohydrate glycogen reserves after around 20–21 miles, they then have to rely on fat as a source of energy in order to carry on running and finish the race. This depletion of carbohydrate stores and the changeover to fat stores takes a little time, affects the running performance and is known as "hitting the wall" (Herbert and Subak-Sharpe, 1995). When this happens the body feels weak and the runner is unable to run at their normal pace.

Fats can be divided into saturated and unsaturated fats, and it is the saturated fats which can have a less than positive health effect on the body, because they can raise cholesterol levels (Vander et al., 1998). Saturated fat is found in full-fat milk, cheese, cream and butter, biscuits, cakes and chocolate. Unsaturated fats can be found naturally in oily fish, such as sardines, fresh tuna and salmon, and are high in omega-3s, which are fatty acids essential to human health, and especially brain and nerve function. White fish such as cod, plaice and haddock are good sources of protein and vitamins A and D, and also contain omega-3 (Nettleton, 1995), but not at the same level as oily fish.

Proteins, although essential, are not an energy source for the sports performer. Proteins are important for muscles, bone and skin regeneration and growth, and are found in meat, eggs and poultry such as chicken and turkey, with turkey being a low fat, high protein food. Proteins are synthesized into essential and non-essential amino acids, 21 of which are needed by the body. The body however can only make 13 of these, and the remaining eight, called the essential amino acids, have to come from animal and plant food. The 13 thirteen amino acids the body can make itself are called the non-essential amino acids (Beashel and Taylor, 1997). The coach can monitor his or her players' daily and weekly dietary intake by using a dietary analysis form, an example of which is given in Appendix 10.

Generally, when fuelling for performance the performer should ensure that glycogen stores are adequate for optimal performance and ideally they should not eat for two hours prior to performance. How to fuel and what to do post-performance is just as important as pre-performance. The first priority post-performance or post-exercise is to replace fluids, which will be looked at in more detail below. Quinn (2008a) suggests that after exercise it is important to consume carbohydrate such as fruit or juice within 15 minutes post-exercise to restore glycogen stores. Research has shown (Ivy *et al.*, 2002; Levenhagen *et al.*, 2002; Zawadzki and Yaspelkis, 1992) that eating 100–200 grams of carbohydrate within two hours of endurance exercise is essential for building adequate glycogen stores for continued training; waiting longer than two hours to eat results in 50 per cent less glycogen stored in the muscle, and combining protein with carbohydrate in the two hours after exercise nearly doubles the insulin response, which results in more stored glycogen.

Water is a crucial constituent for healthy living, and is present in a range of foods and fluids consumed. On a daily basis the human body loses water in urine, sweat and bodily functions, and it needs to be replaced. In sport the body is put under stress and therefore the requirement to hydrate and rehydrate is more important, as dehydration can be a major health issue, especially in hot and humid conditions. "Water loss from the body can be between 2.1 to 2.45 litres per day, and once exercise is under taken, water loss via sweating can be fourteen times greater" (Cole, 2008, p. 1).

There is a wide range of advice available stating when and how much fluid should be consumed pre-, during and post-performance but as a general rule Cole suggests that performers should consume around 500 mls (17 ounces) of fluid two to three hours before exercise, and around 300 mls just before exercise. Carlson (2008) recommends that individuals drink two cups (16 ounces) for every pound lost for the duration of exercise. Although water is a good thirst quencher, sports drinks should be preferred during exercise. Sawka *et al.* (2007, p. 377) suggest that "during exercise, consuming beverages containing electrolytes and carbohydrates can provide benefits over water in certain circumstances, and after exercise the goal is to replace any fluid electrolyte deficit". A range of sports drinks exists, and a range of claims are made regarding the benefits of different types of product. However, sports drinks can be categorized into three types: isotonic, hypotonic and hypertonic. Taranowski (2008) suggests that each has a different function when being absorbed into the body. Isotonic sports drinks have a fluid concentration that is similar to that of blood and are quickly absorbed into the blood stream. Hypotonic sports drinks have a concentration that is lower than the blood and are rapidly absorbed into the blood stream. Hypertonic sports drinks have a higher concentration than the blood and therefore do not absorb into the blood effectively, which slows down the rate at which the stomach empties and reduces the rate of hydration.

If the opportunity arises during natural breaks in performance (time-outs and half-times) fluids should be taken, and post-exercise hydration should aim to correct any fluid loss in order to redress the fluid balance. Fluid loss and replenishment will vary from individual to individual and different formulas based on body weight and length of time exercising purport to inform the individual on how much fluid should be consumed post-performance. The coach, while having a good general knowledge of hydration and rehydration, should seek the advice of a nutritionist to calculate individual differences in fluid consumption and replenishment in a more detailed fashion.

SUMMARY

Knowledge of the structure of human musculoskeletal anatomy is basic to the understanding of human movement and sporting activity. The coach should employ a multi-disciplinary perspective and draw on and have a sound knowledge of a range of disciplines; anatomy and physiology is one of those disciplines.

In order to prepare the performer physically and implement fitness and training programmes, the coach should understand how the body works. The coach should also understand how the body moves and the terms associated with body movement, bone structure and muscle function and composition, even if it is at a very basic level. Knowing how the body works aids understanding in skill delivery, development and execution.

Determining intensity and volume of training is a crucial element in coaching practice and the coach with knowledge of the different energy pathways is able to appreciate the demands and limitations on performers when they are being asked to perform skills and practices. The performer needs to fuel and hydrate sensibly in order to achieve optimal performance and the coach has a significant role to play, educating the performer on when and how to consume which fuels and fluids prior, during and post-performance.

Carbohydrate and fats are the main sources of fuel that are converted into energy in the body. The human body requires water in order to function effectively, and fluid replacement in sport is an important aspect in maintaining optimal sports performance. On a daily basis the human body loses water in urine, sweat and bodily functions, and it needs to be replaced. Water is a good thirst quencher but sports drinks should be preferred for the replacement of lost fluid during exercise because they contain essential metabolites that can aid the glycogen replenishment process.

SEMINAR OR DISCUSSION QUESTIONS

1. Name five terms that are associated with movement of the body.
2. Describe the role of the cardiovascular system.
3. Identify and describe the energy pathways.
4. Describe the role of carbohydrates, fats and proteins.
5. Describe the function of the three main types of sports drink.

KEY TERMS AND DEFINITIONS

- Adenosine tri-phosphate (ATP) – an immediate energy system.
- Aerobic system – with oxygen.
- Anaerobic system – without oxygen.
- Cardiac contractions – initiated by electrical impulse.
- Cardiac muscle – forms the major part of the heart.
- Creatine phosphate – secondary energy system, which is broken down to create ATP.
- Digestion – the breaking down of food in the small and large intestine.
- External respiration – exchange of gases between lungs and the blood.
- Internal respiration – carriage of gases by the blood and the exchange of gases between blood and cells.
- Pulmonary ventilation – breathing.
- Rehydration – effective fluid replenishment.
- Residual volume – air left in the lungs after each breath.

- Skeleton – supports the body by giving it shape, and also provides attachment points for the muscles.
- Smooth muscles – found in layers and form the muscle part of the digestive tract, the bladder, blood vessels and the skin.
- Striated or skeletal muscle – muscle attached to the skeleton.
- Tidal volume – resting air which moves in and out of the lungs in each breath.
- Total lung capacity – the vital capacity plus the residual volume.
- Vital capacity – largest amount of air that can be expelled from the lungs.

WEB LINKS

Energy systems – www.brianmac.co.uk/energy.htm
Heart and lungs – www.smm.org/heart/heart/top.html
Muscles – www.bbc.co.uk/science/humanbody
Nutrition – http://sportsmedicine.about.com/cs/nutrition
Skeletal system – http://42explore.com/skeleton.htm

FURTHER READING

Bartlett, R. (1997). *Introduction to Sports Biomechanics*. E & FN Spon, London.
Beashel, P. and Taylor, J. (1997). *The World of Sport Examined*. Thomas Nelson Publishing, Ontario.
Hardman, A. E. and Stensel, D. J. (2003). *Physical Activity and Health: The Evidence Explained*. Routledge, London.
McKardle, W. D., Katch, F. I. and Katch, V. L. (2007). *Exercise Physiology: Energy, Nutrition and Human Performance*. (6th Ed). Lippincott Williams and Wilkins, London.
McLaughlin, D., Stamford, J. and White, D. (2006). *Instant Notes in Human Physiology*. Routledge, London.
Powers, S. K. and Howley, E. T. (1997). *Exercise Physiology: Theory and Application to Fitness and Performance* (3rd edn). WCB McGraw-Hill, New York.
Shepherd, J. (2006). *The Complete Guide to Sports Training*. A & C Black, London.

Chapter 11

Fundamentals of training and fitness

CHAPTER OBJECTIVES

- Describe the role of the coach in developing fitness training programmes.
- Identify and describe the principles and components of fitness training.
- Identify and describe types of fitness training.
- Describe the integration of multi-directional activities into fitness programmes.
- Provide a case study of a fitness trainer.
- Identify different types of fitness test and when to test.
- Explain strength and conditioning.

THE ROLE OF THE COACH IN DEVELOPING FITNESS TRAINING PROGRAMMES

Fitness programmes and the development of fitness play an essential role in maximizing the effectiveness in performance of athletes, and there is an increasing awareness that fitness has to be monitored methodically and systematically (Wilkinson and Moore, 1995). Many coaches do not have the luxury of being able to employ the services of a fitness trainer to condition their performers pre-, during and post-season, therefore the responsibility may lie with the coach to design and implement a fitness training programme. In these cases the coach should have a good understanding of the principles, components and types of fitness training that are available and which best suit the coach's aims and objectives. Fitness training can be integrated into the overall training programme and should be designed to maximize the physical development of the performers.

When designing a pre-season fitness training programme the coach must ensure that the content, intensity and volume of training is sufficient to prepare the performer to meet the demands of the competitive period, and to maintain fitness levels throughout the season. A consequence of fitness training is that the body goes through physical and psychological adaptations (Galvin and Ledger, 1998) and it takes time for the performer to adapt to the training load; therefore structured, repeated loading and fatiguing fitness sessions are necessary for improvement to occur.

PRINCIPLES AND COMPONENTS OF FITNESS TRAINING

The mnemonic SPORT is widely used for a set of principles to follow in order to train effectively, and should be considered by the coach in designing and implementing a fitness training programme.

S – Specificity. The training needs to be specific to the sport or activity being undertaken. For example, the marathon runner will need to do a lot of endurance training and limited strength training.

P – Progression. Increasing the volume of exercise places added stress on the body and must be done progressively. Increase in volume should not be large enough to cause injury or burnout, but just enough to challenge the mind and body.

O – Overload. The performer needs to overload the body in order to improve fitness. The swimmer who has been swimming six miles twice a week at a regular pace would either increase the distance or raise the swim intensity by completing the six miles in a shorter time, or swimming three times a week.

R – Reversibility. Ceasing training can have reversing effects. For example, it takes around three to four weeks to lose physical conditioning, and aerobic fitness is lost quicker than anaerobic fitness. The coach must therefore consider that during recovery periods some physical activity is continued to maintain a level of fitness.

T – Tedium – the coach should ensure that the training programme includes a variety of training methods in order to maintain the motivational levels of the performer(s) and ensure that they do not become bored.

(Adapted from Beashel and Taylor, 1997; Galvin and Ledger, 1998; Lee, 1993)

When designing fitness training programmes the coach must be able to identify the fitness components that make up the physical demands of the sport and train them accordingly. The components to be trained will depend on the nature and demands of the sport, e.g. the fitness components to be trained for a table tennis player will differ significantly to those of a weightlifter. The following are fitness components that can be developed in a fitness training programme:

- Aerobic endurance – involves whole body exercise for a prolonged period of time, continuously.
- Explosive power – the ability to exert maximum muscular contraction instantly in an explosive burst of movements; the two components of power are strength and speed.
- Speed – ability to move the body and body parts quickly in time, space and over distance.
- Muscular endurance – ability to work a muscle or muscle groups intensively for a prolonged period of time.
- Flexibility – the ability to achieve an extended range of motion in the muscles and joints.

(Foran, 2001).

Although not fitness components, the following are abilities that can also be trained:

- Agility – the ability to change direction at speed.
- Balance – ability to control the body's position while either stationary or moving and can

be divided into static balance, which is seen in gymnasts, and dynamic balance, which is seen in water skiers, wake boarders and windsurfers.

■ Coordination – an organized, economic and fluent working of body parts such as running, jumping, kicking, catching and throwing.

TYPES OF FITNESS TRAINING

Different types of fitness training exist that can enhance development of the components of fitness training. In many sports an integrative approach is required, where the coach can utilize a series of types of fitness training in order to address the components and physical demands of the sport. Alternatively, there may be a requirement to concentrate on one component for a performer who is returning from injury.

Different types of fitness training include continuous, Fartlek, interval, weight and plyometric training (Moran and McGlynn, 1997). Continuous training is exercising at a steady rate and is a good way for an athlete to build up their cardiovascular endurance fitness. This type of training suits long distance runners because their endurance levels will increase, and it mimics the competitive environment in which they race in. Fartlek training is a continuous form of training in which the aerobic and anaerobic systems are put under stress by varying speed and intensity (Sandrock, 2000). Fartlek training is generally associated with running, but can include almost any kind of exercise including cycling, rowing or swimming. Interval training involves the performer "interspersing heavy periods of intense activity with recovery periods of slower activity" (Billat, 2001, p. 14), which may include either a passive or active recovery (Shepherd, 2006). The swimmer may swim hard and fast over a distance up to one kilometre and then have a recovery period of a slower swim of around two hundred metres and then swim hard and fast again for another kilometre. During the fast swim period, lactic acid is produced and a state of oxygen debt is reached. During the interval (recovery period), the heart and lungs are still stimulated as they try to pay back the debt by supplying oxygen to help break down the lactates (Maglischo, 2003).

The stresses put upon the body cause an adaptation and strengthening of the heart muscles and improved oxygen uptake, which leads to improved performance, in particular within the cardiovascular system (Quinn, 2008b). Weight training must be designed to be specific to the type of strength and sport. The coach should have knowledge of the types of muscular activity associated with the particular sport, the movement pattern involved and the type of strength required. Exercises should be identified that will produce the desired development of the performer's strength.

Plyometric training is effective for improving explosive power. Developing the lower limb major muscle groups using plyometrics improves the body's capability to allow faster and more powerful changes and enables efficient transfer of energy in the direction of movement (Chu, 1998), and is used to enable both strength development and explosive power (Gordon, 2009). As a word of caution for coaches, it is recommended that the coach ensures that they are at least four to six weeks into a fitness training programme before implementing plyometrics training because it involves a lot of leaping, jumping and bounding. Significant strain is placed on the insertion muscles, tendons and joints in the ankles, knees and hips when carrying out this training method and there could be a potential for injury if the performer is not fully warmed up and muscle strength has not been developed.

INTEGRATION OF MULTI-DIRECTIONAL ACTIVITIES INTO FITNESS TRAINING PROGRAMMES

Coaches of many sports such as cricket, field hockey, soccer and tennis are now beginning to integrate multi-directional activities into their fitness training programmes, rather than just implementing a running and circuit training programme which for many performers is just a chore pre-season. Multi-directional fitness training utilizes ladders, hurdles, cones and a variety of other equipment in order to develop a range of motor skills such as agility, balance, coordination, quickness and speed. For this reason, coaches are beginning to understand that carrying out multi-directional activities that are specific to the demands and the nature of their sport can be a more effective training method.

The coach does not require a large space to deliver a multi-directional fitness training session; all that is required is hurdles, ladders and cones, and a creative mind to ensure variability of practice throughout the fitness training programme. The primary focus for these sessions is quality of movement, not quantity; however, with a well-structured session the performers actually do cover a lot of ground which, on top of developing a range of fundamental motor skills, enhances their aerobic capacity and keeps them interested and motivated. This would probably not be the case if they were expected to just go on a three-mile run and come back to do some circuit training.

The coach can also combine the development of fundamental motor skills with technical skills by adding a stick, racket or ball, depending on the nature of the sport. For example, the coach may instruct his tennis player to conduct a series of lateral explosive movements left, right, forwards and backwards while being thrown a tennis ball, which would mimic the player having to move around the court to execute a service return. Running and circuit training does have its place, but the coach should be creative in implementing sports specific activities that keep the performer interested and have more relation to the demands of the sport that is being trained for.

Case study 11.1 – The role of the fitness trainer

Paul has been a professional fitness trainer for eight years, and has had a range of clients, such as British power lifters, rugby players, volleyball players, male and female National League field hockey players; and an international (England) field hockey player. When Paul started out as a professional fitness trainer his clients ranged from individuals who wanted to lose weight to individuals who just wanted to improve fitness. Paul also conducts courses in core stability and is a SAQ® tutor and trainer; currently he is an associate lecturer and fitness consultant at a UK university and a local field hockey club.

When working with individual clients Paul always draws up an Individual Fitness Plan. With a plan that is easy to follow, Paul is able to monitor his client or performer, and the plan also becomes a self-motivator for the client. These plans can also be reviewed after around three months in conjunction with the client in order for the client to monitor progress and if any changes are required then the plan can be adapted to suit the needs of the client.

When working with a team a generic plan is produced that is split into two main programmes; an 8-to-12-week pre-season training programme and an in-season training programme. The content of the pre-season programme consists of aerobic fitness, strength, endurance, agility, balance and coordination training. The in-season programme consists mainly of sport-specific training, including the movement patterns of the sport, agility training and individual aerobic and strength training programmes. Major emphasis is also placed on injury prevention by using core stability training techniques.

When initially assessing his performers, Paul uses fitness testing techniques which provide a baseline measure to compare later results of tests that may be administered during the in-season. Paul has developed a sport-specific (field hockey) test that he feels is a more reliable predictor of sport-specific fitness. This test is a maximum effort test, which operates on a running clock and is only stopped when the test is over. The test is deemed over if the performer completes it in 12 minutes or less; the quicker the time, the fitter the performer. Although this test is similar to the Cooper Run, Paul's test is a maximum test and has recovery periods incorporated within it, which mimics the nature and demands of field hockey. Paul uses fitness-assessment records to monitor and record fitness performance, and feels that they are more useful to the person who wants to lose weight because the record can be used as a motivational and goal-setting tool.

Paul feels that performer fitness-assessment records are not so important in a team environment and that fitness trainers should guard against the performer's perception bias. Specifically, the performer may not put in his or her best effort in the pre-season baseline test, knowing that when they are re-tested in a couple of months they will perform better, which could be viewed as a distorted measure of fitness. The performer is leading the fitness trainer or coach to believe that they have improved their fitness when in reality they have not. Paul's fitness training philosophy centres on the belief that if the performer turns up to a fitness training session they are there to train. Moreover, the effort that the performer puts in will reap fitness and sports performance benefits in the long term, and at the same time the performer will achieve his or her goals.

When Paul designs and implements fitness training programmes he also takes into account hydration and nutritional requirements, and feels that it is important to know his client's or team's medical history, which will include injury history, any recent surgery and any other medical conditions that may impact upon fitness testing and physical conditioning. A further consideration for Paul is the possible referral of his performers to a physician prior to them participating in a fitness programme.

FITNESS TESTING

Today's modern coach should be capable of administering, recording and analysing fitness test results to feedback to the performer, and tests can be carried out either in a laboratory or in the field setting. Laboratory testing has an advantage over field-based fitness testing because it is governed by strict testing protocols that have been robustly tested over time. Alternatively, field-based fitness testing is easy to implement and is time- and cost-effective in terms of facilities and equipment (Wilkinson and Moore, 1995).

There are a number of tests available that are adequate for the coach to use in the field, but they have to be administered effectively in order to get as accurate results as possible. There are also a number of reasons why the coach may want to test the fitness of their performer(s), and the coach should explain fully to the performers the reasons why they are being tested in order to fully engage them in the process. The reasons for administering fitness tests may be to determine a baseline measure so that fitness can be monitored throughout the season; to help performers set fitness goals for the season; to allow assessment of a training programme; to identify areas of perceived need in a performer's fitness (Caplan and Adams, 2007); and to investigate the fitness requirements of a particular position in a team game. The tests can be used as a feedback tool on a performer's fitness progress since returning from injury and can possibly contribute towards a talent identification profile, which can be used for selection purposes (Wilkinson and Moore, 1995). However, caution must be exercised when using fitness assessments as a selection tool as it is only one part of overall sports performance.

A fitness test will only give information on one fitness component and therefore the type of test to administer will be dependent on the sport and which fitness components are important in the sport. In order to select an appropriate test the coach can construct a fitness profile identifying the fitness components and rating the relative importance of each component on a scale from one to five. Once this has been achieved the coach can select the appropriate test designed to assess the identified fitness component. An example of a blank fitness profile is given in Appendix 11. Once the coach knows which fitness component they are testing and with what test, they will need to decide *when* to test. The coach should integrate a fitness training programme into the overall season plan, and within that plan there will be opportunities to identify appropriate points in the plan to conduct fitness testing.

Generally, testing takes place in the pre-season phase of the training programme and at specific points during the season, which might be after a recovery period or for a player returning from injury. The coach should not test for "testing's sake", testing must be objective and have value. Prior to actually administering the test the coach should arrive at the venue early to set up any equipment, such as cones and the working area, and also consider the surface being used. During the summer many sand-based AstroTurfs become very dry, and sometimes slips occur because the performer is unable to get sufficient grip on the dry sand surface, which impacts upon the performer's carrying out the test effectively and possibly distorting the time taken to do the test.

It is essential the coach ensures that the performers carry out a full warm-up prior to the test and familiarizes the performers with the test. They also must provide consent forms for those performers undertaking the test who are under eighteen years of age, ensure that external motivational factors are limited (other participants observing the test) and that the test procedures are adhered to. The measuring equipment that is used must be accurate and reliable (Rikli and Jones, 2001) and an assistant should be present to assist with the scoring. A further important consideration in field-based fitness testing is to ensure that when re-testing, the test is administered under the same conditions.

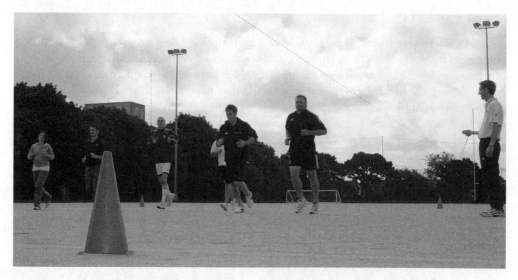

Photo 11.1 A coach conducting a fitness test.

Kilgore and Touchberry (2007) suggest a series of easy-to-administer tests which are able to test the following fitness components in the field-based setting:

- Aerobic endurance – the multi-stage fitness test, the Harvard step test, the Cooper 12-minute run, a performance timed run over 1.5 miles.
- Strength – one-repetition max. bench press or ten-repetition max. leg press.
- Muscular power – standing vertical jump, standing broad jump and Magaria staircase test.
- Explosive speed – timed sprint test.
- Strength (muscular endurance) – sit-ups, press-ups and repeated sprints
- Flexibility – sit and reach tests.

Although agility, balance and coordination are not fitness components the following tests can also be used:

- Agility – the Illinois agility test.
- Balance – the stork stand.
- Coordination – the alternate wall toss test.

(Beashel and Taylor, 1997; Mackenzie, 2008a)

Tables 11.1 and 11.2 respectively show a male field hockey team's Illinois agility and sprint test scores (in seconds) pre-season and at a later point in the season.

STRENGTH AND CONDITIONING

The basic aspects of strength and conditioning training involve overloading various muscle groups by using a range of different exercises, repetitions and sets at different levels of force to facilitate changes in strength endurance (Brewer, 2005). Strength and conditioning is not bodybuilding. Bodybuilding is a sport in which the goal is to increase muscle size and definition, it does increase the endurance of muscle, but nowhere near as much as strength and

Table 11.1 *Male field hockey players' Illinois agility test results (in seconds)*

Player	Age	Pre-	Post-
1	22	17.87	17.11
2	24	15.62	16.02
3	29	18.21	17.05
4	26	16.13	16.09
5	26	16.45	16.32
6	25	15.29	16.04
7	18	17.22	16.82
8	31	18.59	17.66
9	18	18.24	16.98
10	22	17.11	16.86
11	20	16.02	16.22
12	21	16.77	16.01

Table 11.2 Male field hockey players' sprint test results (in seconds)

Player	Age	10 metres		20 metres		40 metres	
		Pre	Post	Pre	Post	Pre	Post
1	22	2.61	2.63	4.16	4.20	5.11	5.08
2	24	2.72	2.69	4.21	4.17	5.02	5.13
3	29	2.31	2.39	3.98	4.07	5.31	5.29
4	26	2.58	2.99	4.22	4.14	5.34	5.37
5	31	2.71	3.17	4.92	4.51	5.39	5.42
6	25	2.89	3.09	4.77	4.62	5.41	5.47
7	18	2.76	2.81	3.90	4.01	5.19	5.23
8	26	2.64	2.94	4.29	4.13	5.22	5.19
9	18	2.58	2.98	4.08	4.19	5.37	5.31
10	22	2.92	3.41	4.59	4.31	5.72	5.60
11	20	2.97	3.21	4.47	4.28	5.61	5.58
12	21	2.86	3.07	4.62	4.23	5.14	5.20

conditioning. Bodybuilders compete in bodybuilding competitions, and use specific principles and methods of strength and conditioning training, such as light or heavy weights, slow or fast reps and long or short workouts to maximize muscular size. They develop extremely low levels of body fat (Venuto, 2009) and their only focus is on how they look on stage in a contest.

In contrast, most strength and conditioning coaches train to improve strength and endurance while not focusing too much on reducing body fat and the cosmetics of muscle definition. Strength and conditioning coaches tend to focus on foundation strength, and in comparison bodybuilders use exercises to enhance muscular definition which can be viewed as visually artistic. The specific combinations of exercises depend on the requirements and purpose of the individual carrying out the strength and conditioning programme, and the sport in which they are participating. For example, a javelin thrower returning from a serious shoulder injury may be provided with a specific strength and conditioning programme to redevelop and strengthen the arm and shoulder muscles so that full training can be resumed and he or she can return to competition.

In strength and conditioning training programmes, sets with fewer repetitions can be performed using more force to increase strength, but these have can impact on endurance. Strength and conditioning training also requires the use of good form and the performing of the movements with the appropriate muscle group(s) (Baechle and Earle, 2000). If during the training set the muscle focused on is not being worked at its optimum threshold and form is not good, this can result in injury and the muscle not gaining in strength.

Strength and conditioning programmes have a range of other benefits other than improving strength endurance, such as increased muscle mass, increased tendon and ligament strength and elasticity, increased bone density and strength, increased flexibility and body definition and increased metabolic rate and postural support (Brewer, 2005). While coaches regularly develop and implement fitness training programmes, it is recommended that if there is a specific requirement for a strength and conditioning programme that the coach seeks advice from a qualified strength and conditioning coach.

SUMMARY

Fitness programmes and the development of fitness play an essential role in maximizing the effectiveness in performance of athletes, and there is an increasing awareness that fitness has to be monitored methodically and systematically (Wilkinson and Moore, 1995). Coaches are finding that they are more involved in developing and implementing fitness training programmes in a range of environments for the benefit of their performers.

Fitness training can be integrated into the overall training programme and should be designed to maximize the physical development of the performers. On implementation of the programme specific principles should be accounted for that enable the efficient and successful delivery of the programme. Initially, the coach should identify the fitness components that make up the demands of their particular sport and then identify which type of fitness training is appropriate to implement. For example, if the sport is associated with high levels of aerobic endurance then continuous training would be the preferred method of training.

The coach needs a set of principles to follow in order to train effectively, and the SPORT mnemonic (Specificity, Progression, Overload, Reversibility and Tedium) is a recommended way to train the performer.

In order to monitor fitness levels the coach can implement a range of fitness tests that assess the different fitness components and others exist for assessing agility, balance and coordination. Many sports are integrating multi-directional activities into their fitness training programmes, and ladders, cones and a range of other specialist equipment is becoming commonplace in pre-season fitness training sessions.

Strength and conditioning programmes are also being utilized and implemented by coaches. Strength and conditioning differentiates itself from bodybuilding in that it concentrates on strength endurance training rather than building muscle mass and definition for specific bodybuilding competitions.

SEMINAR OR DISCUSSION QUESTIONS

1. Highlight the fitness components in a sport of your choice and identify which type of training would be appropriate to train the performer.
2. After highlighting the fitness components and type of training, identify which test would be appropriate to assess the particular fitness component(s).

KEY TERMS AND DEFINITIONS

- Fitness component – a specific demand of a sport (e.g. aerobic endurance).
- Fitness training – a process by which the performer trains specific components that make up the demands of a sport.
- Fitness testing – process by which the coach can assess and monitor a performer's fitness levels.
- Multi-directional training – development of a range of biomotor skills such as agility, balance, coordination, quickness and speed.

- Pre-conditioning – training to train.
- SPORT – a mnemonic for a set of principles to follow in order to train effectively.
- Strength and conditioning – a training method than concentrates on developing strength endurance.

WEB LINKS

Fitness tests – www.sport-fitness-advisor.com/fitnesstests.html
Fitness training – www.netfit.co.uk/wkmen.htm
          – www.pponline.co.uk
Strength and conditioning – www.uksca.org.uk

FURTHER READING

Beashel, P. and Taylor, J. (1997). *The World of Sport Examined*. Thomas and Nelson Publishing, Ontario.

Brewer, C. (2005). *Strength and Conditioning for Games Players*. Coachwise/SportsCoachUK, Leeds.

Shepherd, J. (2006). *The Complete Guide to Sports Training*. A & C Black, London.

Wilkinson, D. and Moore, P. (1995). *Measuring Performance: A Guide to Field Based Fitness Testing*. National Coaching Foundation, Leeds.

Winter, E. R. C., Jones, A. M., Davison, R., Bromley, P. and Mercer, T. (2006). *Sport and Exercise Physiology Testing Guidelines* (Vols I and II). Routledge, London.

Chapter 12

Injury prevention

CHAPTER OBJECTIVES

■ Describe the nature of injury.
■ Describe and explain the principles of warming up and cooling down.
■ Explain the concept of the "warm-up decrement".
■ Highlight developments in injury prevention.

THE NATURE OF INJURY

Unfortunately, sport and injury sometimes go hand in hand and therefore the coach should have at least some basic knowledge of how injuries occur and how to prevent them. If the coach follows health and safety guidelines, educates and prepares his or her performers appropriately and constructs a carefully planned training programme, then the potential for injury can be minimized. Sports scientists and coaches have recently developed the concept of "pre-conditioning" (pre-training) as a means of reducing injury and improving sports performance (Shepherd, 2006). Pre-conditioning means "training to train" and the focus is placed on protecting and strengthening the body parts which are susceptible to injury.

Injuries can come in many forms, such as internal injuries, impact, environmental and over-use injuries (Eustice and Eustice, 2006). Internal injuries are the result of stresses on joints, ligaments, tendons or muscles and may be caused by over-extension or over-rotation of a joint. Impact injuries are the result of direct contact with an opponent or piece of equipment, such as an uppercut in boxing, a tackle in rugby, or being struck with a hockey stick or a cricket ball and can cause bone fractures, bruising or a dislocation. Environmental injuries are the result of exercising or performing in extreme weather conditions and can cause further medical complications such as dehydration, heat stroke or hypothermia.

Over-use injuries are the result of using a specific body part repetitively for a prolonged period of time. Excessive and repeated stress placed on joints and tendons can reduce the effective functioning of joints and body parts and cause tendonitis or shin splints. For example, the tennis player may suffer from tendonitis in the elbow through playing a range of service returns over a long period of time. Or the long distance runner who continually trains on roads may suffer from shin splints.

Acute injuries are severe and intense, and are usually to the joints, muscles, tendons and ligaments. They can cause bleeding, swelling and pain. "Female athletes are at four to seven times greater risk of anterior cruciate ligament injury than males playing at similar levels in the same sports, because of gender differences in hip and limb alignment, which can lead to increased knee joint torsion in women" (Shepherd, 2006, p. 33). Chronic injuries are those that are long-lasting and may be over-use injuries such as the discus thrower having back and shoulder problems after continual throwing and trunk rotation over a long period of time.

Many athletes are seen by a physiotherapist or sports therapist following injury. However, increasingly these professionals are seeing the performer prior to any injury occurring as a preventative measure and are providing screening sessions (Rose and Everard, 2007). The screening sessions are designed to identify any pre-existing joint or ligament weaknesses or muscle imbalances, and then treatment is administered accordingly to prevent any further problems. Moreover, these screening sessions help highlight problems such as muscle tightness and joint mobility that result from the stresses of training and competition. The coach is well placed to educate his or her performers, and an important part of injury prevention is not letting a minor strain develop into something more serious, which would inhibit the recovery process and consequently prevent the performer from continuing training.

The coach also has a responsibility not to put pressure on the performer to return to training and competition before they are fit to do so. Moreover, many injuries occur because the performer has either not warmed up or cooled down properly; therefore the importance of carrying out these two practices cannot be stressed enough.

WARMING UP AND COOLING DOWN

Developing a structured warm-up for performers is a key coaching role, and an important factor in the prevention of injury. A warm-up should not only be used before the start of an activity, but also if there are prolonged breaks in activity or performance. A range of benefits is associated with a warm-up which include:

- increased speed of contraction and relaxation of warmed muscles
- greater economy of movement because of lowered viscous resistance within warmed muscles
- facilitated oxygen utilization by warmed muscles, because haemoglobin releases oxygen more readily at higher muscle temperatures
- facilitated nerve transmission and muscle metabolism at higher temperatures
- increased blood flow through active tissues
- increased arousal and focusing of attention
- reduces muscle stiffness.

(Adapted from Mackenzie, 2008 and Quinn, 2008c)

Muscle stiffness is thought to be directly related to muscle injury, therefore a warm-up should be aimed at reducing muscle stiffness (Herbert and Gabriel, 2002), be sport-specific and not just a series of stretches. In 2004 Stephen Thacker, Director of the Epidemiology Program Office at the Centers for Disease Control and Prevention (CDC) in Atlanta, USA, reviewed more than 350 articles on stretching and warm-up and concluded that there was insufficient evidence to support the effectiveness of stretching. Moreover, studies (Herbert and Gabriel, 2002; Shrier, 1999) have found little evidence to support injury prevention by static stretching prior to or after performance, and have suggested that static stretching may even negatively affect performance. However, in sports such as gymnastics regular stretching does increase static flexibility, where the normal range of motion of the muscles is exceeded (Groner, 2004).

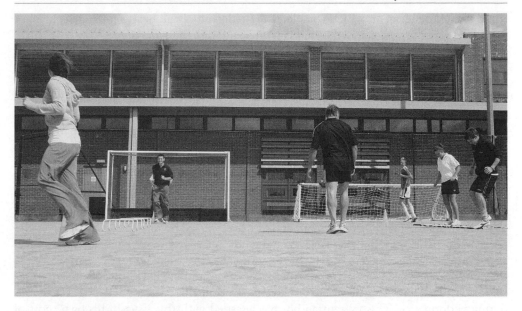

Photo 12.1 A coach conducting a warm-up.

Many sports are now integrating sport-specific, multi-directional, dynamic stretching activities that mimic the actions of the sport being performed. Speed, Agility and Quickness (SAQ®, 2003) principles such as Dynamic Flex® stretching, which is moving while stretching (i.e. arm swings, hip and knee rotations, toe raises while walking), and Dynamic Flex® warm-ups are being implemented into many pre-training and pre-competition routines. Olympic gold medal winner and world champion triple jumper Jonathan Edwards in an interview for a UK newspaper indicated that he had changed his warm-up a number of years ago, from one that incorporated a series of static movements to one that works through a whole range of movements (Pearson, 2004). Many sports are now seeing the benefits of integrating these types of warm-ups into their pre-training and pre-competition routines.

Cooling down properly is as equally important as warming up, and a proper cool-down should be conducted post-performance. A cool-down aids in the following:

- dissipation of waste products in the muscles (lactic acid)
- reduces the potential for delayed onset of muscle soreness (DOMS)
- reduces levels of adrenaline in the blood
- reduces heart rate and blood flow
- returns the body to a relaxed state.

(The Stretching Institute, 2008)

Gupta *et al.* (1996) propose that the cool-down should consist of two parts; the sport-specific activity and static stretching. The sport-specific activity gradually reduces the heart rate and blood flow and is an active recovery element. Gupta *et al.* go on to suggest that an active type of recovery is the best way of enhancing lactate removal after exercise.

The Dynamic Flex® (Pearson, 2004) cool-down would be an appropriate active recovery, sport-specific activity to carry out, using the same types of movement patterns as the Dynamic Flex ® warm-up but at a much slower pace. The second part of the cool-down would be the static stretching element, which completes the reducing of the heart rate and removal of metabolic waste products, inducing muscular relaxation at the same time.

THE WARM-UP DECREMENT

It is important for the coach to understand the concept of the warm-up decrement in the context of warming up and cooling down, and the impact it can have on breaks in performance. Sports which have "rolling" substitutions such as field hockey are particularly relevant to this issue. Players come off for a break and then after a short period of time return to the game, and this can happen as many as four or five times in a game of field hockey, or more if the game is being played in particularly hot and humid conditions.

During this period of rest there is a reduction in performance attention levels (Nacson and Schmidt, 1971) and attention, arousal and warm-up levels are not at the same level as when initiating performance (Schmidt and Lee, 1999). The focus is on listening to the coach's instructions so the body begins cooling down, the end result being a reduced level of performance. The problem is that when performance is resumed it takes a period of time to get back to the same levels as when performance was initiated. This has implications for some sports that have long half-time breaks, excessive time-out periods and long rest periods during performance. This present author has wrestled with this issue in his own sport of field hockey, and has wanted to reduce the amount of time the coach provides performance instructional feedback to a minimum in the ten-minute break, down to five minutes. For the remaining five minutes a mini warm-up could be conducted in order to re-energize the performers, which would hopefully limit the effects of the warm-up decrement. The major issue however, is getting the players to buy into the idea, and for coaches to be able to reduce their half-time team talk to a few basic instructions and feedback. This would require a major shift in the emphasis of thinking in coaching practice.

DEVELOPMENTS IN INJURY PREVENTION

Current thinking has advanced in the prevention of injury and enhancing the recovery process for the performer. One of the now most widely used methods is the ice bath, which reportedly enhances the body's natural recovery process (Lee, 2008; Smith, 2008) and is used predominantly in high impact sports such boxing and rugby. However, the method is increasingly being used in a range of sports. Although many performers and coaches are nothing but positive about the effects of an ice bath on recovery, there are conflicting views in the academic literature regarding its efficacy, with Eston and Peters (1999) and Sellwood et al. (2007) suggesting that they are of no use. Another treatment that has been developed to enhance the recovery process is alternating hot and cold water immersion. However, Cochrane (2003, p. 26) suggests that "more research is needed before conclusions can be drawn on whether alternating hot–cold water immersion improves recuperation and influences the physiological changes that characterises post exercise recovery".

Another method which is not so much for enhancing the recovery process and preventing injury but for regulating the body's core temperature is pre-cooling. This process is used in a high temperature or high humidity environment in order to regulate the body's core temperature so that the performer can function and execute performance without over-heating. Paula Radcliffe, the UK marathon runner, wore an ice jacket prior to starting the women's marathon event in the 2004 Athens Olympiad in order to keep her core temperature as normal as possible in heat conditions that would reach 35 degrees Celsius during the race.

During the 2008 Beijing Olympic Games it was evident that some athletes were wearing ice jackets when being interviewed post-competition, in order to return their body's core temperature to normal levels.

SUMMARY

The coach should have at least some basic knowledge of how injuries occur and how to prevent them. Different types of injuries exist, such as internal, impact, environmental, over-use, acute and chronic injuries. Increasingly physiotherapists and sports therapists are seeing the performer prior to any injury as a preventative measure and providing screening and MOT sessions. The screening sessions are designed to identify any pre-existing joint or ligament weaknesses or muscle imbalances, and then treatment is administered accordingly to prevent any further problems. The MOT is designed to help address problems such as muscle tightness and joint mobility that result from the stresses of training and competition.

The coach has a responsibility not to put pressure on the performer to return to training and competition before they are fit to do so. Many injuries occur because the performer has either not warmed up or cooled down properly; therefore the importance of carrying out these two practices cannot be stressed enough. The warm-up should be sport-specific – gone are the days when the performers went for a jog then carried out some random static (passive) stretching. In fact, research has shown that static stretching is ineffectual and may even negatively affect performance. Coaches are now integrating sport-specific, multi-directional, dynamic stretching activities into warm-ups. This type of activity mimics the actions of the sport being performed, and coaches and performers are now seeing the benefits of integrating these types of warm-ups into their pre-training and pre-competition routines.

Cooling down properly is as important as warming up, and a proper cool-down should be conducted post-performance. The cool-down returns the body to a relaxed state and removes waste products (lactic acid) from the muscles, reducing the potential for DOMS.

The warm-up decrement is a neuropsychophysiological phenomenon causing sporting performance to decrease following a period of rest, e.g. half-time in soccer, rugby or field hockey. Current thinking has advanced in the prevention of injury and enhancing the recovery process for the performer. Ice baths and hot and cold water immersion techniques are being used in order to further enhance the recovery of a performer.

SEMINAR OR DISCUSSION QUESTIONS

1. Design a dynamic warm-up in a sport of your choice.
2. Explain the concept of the warm-up decrement.

KEY TERMS AND DEFINITIONS

■   Acute injuries – severe and intense injuries.
■   Chronic injuries – long-lasting injuries.

- DOMS – delayed onset muscle soreness.
- Dynamic Flex® – warm-up and cool-down process, which incorporates multi-directional movement while stretching.
- Dynamic stretching – moving while stretching.
- Environmental injuries – result of exercising or performing in extreme weather conditions.
- Impact injuries – result of direct contact with an opponent or piece of equipment.
- Internal injuries – result of stresses on joints, ligaments, tendons or muscles.
- Over-use injuries – result of using a specific body part repetitively.
- Pre-cooling – a process that helps regulate the body's core temperature.
- Warm-up decrement – following a period of rest, sports performance will decrease temporarily.

WEB LINKS

British Chiropractic Association – www.chiropractic-uk.co.uk
Chartered Society of Physiotherapy – www.csp.org.uk
General Osteopathic Council – www.osteopathy.org.uk
Warming up and cooling down – www.brianmac.co.uk

FURTHER READING

Brown, L. E and Ferrigno, V. A. (2005). *Training for Speed, Agility and Quickness* (2nd edn). Human Kinetics, Champaign, IL.
Frederick, A. M. and Frederick, C. (2006). *Stretch to Win*. Coachwise/SportsCoachUK, Leeds.
Pearson, A. (2004). *Dynamic Flexibility: Warming up on the Move*. A & C Black, London.
Shepherd, J. (2006). *The Complete Guide to Sports Training*. A & C Black, London.

Psychology, performance analysis and the role of the coach

INTRODUCTION

Part 5 outlines the role of the coach in utilizing sports psychology and taking a skill acquisition approach in their coaching, as well as discussing the use of technology for performance analysis and basic biomechanics.

Chapter 13 provides a case study of a practising accredited sports psychologist and his role in working with coaches. It outlines mental skills such as confidence enhancement, concentration, motivation, anxiety and anxiety reduction, arousal reduction and inducing arousal, imagery, goal-setting and utilization of pre-performance routines, and how the coach can integrate these into coaching practice.

Chapter 14 highlights the role of the coach in applying skill acquisition principles and differentiates between skill and ability before examining the processes by which the performer learns and the strategies by which the coach can facilitate these processes. A basic understanding of the information processing approach compared to the ecological approach to coaching will be provided, and the processes of feedback, selective attention, decision making, anticipation, reaction time and the role of memory will be comprehensively examined. Differing types of practice, such as random, blocked, variable, massed, distributed and deliberate practice will be explored, with practical examples of how each can be structured in a coaching environment in order to facilitate effective performer learning.

In Chapter 15 basic biomechanics are outlined in a coach-friendly manner, while at the same time providing the necessary information to enable the coach to understand and apply the fundamental concepts of physics and mechanics to the way in which the human body moves. Also in Chapter 15 basic types of software and technological tools, such as digital versatile cameras (DVCs) that are available to the coach are identified, as well as advances in technology that are currently being used to support the coach in performance analysis. The use of pen and paper notational analysis is examined, with examples of how this concept can be utilized effectively in the coaching environment. At the end of the chapter suggested seminar or discussion questions are provided, along with key terms and definitions. Web links and suggested further reading are also provided if more information or further research is required.

Chapter 13

Psychology and the coach

⚡

CHAPTER OBJECTIVES

■ Identify the role of the sports psychologist in supporting the coach.
■ Provide a case study of the sports psychologist and the coach.
■ Explain confidence and identify confidence enhancement strategies.
■ Explain concentration and identify concentration strategies.
■ Explain motivation and how to develop a motivational climate.
■ Explain anxiety and identify anxiety reduction strategies.
■ Explain arousal and identify arousal reducing and inducement techniques.
■ Explain imagery and identify imagery techniques.
■ Explain and identify pre-performance routines.
■ Explain goal setting and identify the goal setting process.

THE ROLE OF THE SPORTS PSYCHOLOGIST

Psychologists function in a range of sub-disciplines including educational, clinical, counselling, research and applied psychology. The sports psychologist falls into one of three main categories: educational, research or applied. "Sports psychology is a science in which the principles of psychology are applied in a sport or exercise setting, and are often applied to enhance sport and exercise performance" (Cox, 1998, p. 4).

In the USA sports psychology has been regulated and professionalized for many years, whereas organizations in the UK such as the British Psychological Society (BPS) and British Association of Sport and Exercise Sciences (BASES) are still developing processes whereby those wishing to become sports psychologists can be accredited and certified competent to practice. These processes are soon to become more robust because under current law anyone can claim to be a psychologist and offer services to the public, irrespective of their training or experience.

The BPS has sought public protection and now the UK government wants to regulate the profession through the Health Professions Council (HPC). One of the effects of the proposed legislation will be that nobody will be able to call themselves a sports psychologist unless they are registered with the HPC, which requires evidence of a formal qualification and continued practice or CPD. In essence, when the legislation is introduced no unqualified coach will be able to describe themselves as a "sports psychologist" (SportsCoachUK, 2008g).

It is interesting that while some coaches will seek the help of a fitness trainer to support them in developing fitness training programmes, there is still reticence among coaches to approach a sports psychologist for support in developing mental skills training programmes. Arguably, this could be partly due to coaches being more comfortable in dealing with technical and strategic delivery and fitness training and partly due to a lack of understanding of what the roles of sports psychology and the sports psychologist are (Winstone, 2007).

It is crucial that the coach understands that the sports psychologist should be utilized in a supporting role and that they are not there to undermine the coach, because the coach has the ultimate responsibility of performance outcomes. However, if the coach does require the services of a sports psychologist they should contact BASES or the BPS who will be able to provide details of accredited practitioners.

Case study 13.1 – The sports psychologist and the coach

Tim is a BASES accredited sports psychologist who has been practising for nineteen years, and a reader in Sports Psychology at a UK university. Tim has provided sports science support (sports psychology) to the following sports: athletics, boxing, hockey, ice skating, judo, real tennis, sailing, squash, swimming, table tennis and tennis.

Tim identifies the fact that different approaches are needed when working with individuals in comparison to working with team sports. When providing support in a team environment, most of the interventions that are put in place centre on teamwork, cohesiveness, role clarity, group work and squad ethics and values. Individual sports performers require more performance enhancement interventions, such as standard mental skills, e.g. concentration strategies, confidence enhancement and anxiety reduction.

In his early days of practising Tim found that performers were not interested in having the coach involved when requesting the services of a sports psychologist. This is now rare, and the process is becoming more integrated into the coach's role, with the coach understanding how they and the performer can collaborate together. When working with a new coach Tim first gains their trust and suggests that sports psychology can be complementary to the coaching process rather than contradictory. The working relationship between the sports psychologist and the coach varies, and is dependent on the coach's openness. Some coaches look to work with the sports psychologist themselves more than having the sports psychologist work with the performer(s), because the coach is perhaps looking to improve his or her coaching and glean information and implement ideas used by the sports psychologist for themselves and the performer.

Tim suggests that a good coach is a good sports psychologist, but they probably do not recognize that themselves, and there are limits to what a coach is able to do. The good coach is able to remind and reinforce simple and concrete strategies that the sports psychologist has originally implemented, as the coach in reality has more contact with the performer. However, it can be frustrating at times because the delivery of interventions by the sports psychologist can be fragmented, and they are not able to see the whole process through. Therefore it is important to work *through* coaches, so that regular access can be obtained to the performer. This means that the whole process can be seen through from initial assessment to a reflect and review of interventions and strategies put in place.

A range of different interventions can be put in place to support the performer which are generally sport-dependent, and coaches generally request interventions on the key areas that are most relevant to their sport and has the biggest demand. For example, the key intervention that is asked for in boxing is concentration improvement, in sailing it is decision making and in swimming its motivation work that is most commonly requested.

If coaches require an educational awareness session it will generally be on a specific topic, e.g. goal setting. The most commonly requested specific interventions by most performers are emotional control, confidence enhancement and concentration. Coaches have also requested specific support for themselves in terms of dealing with conflict, motivating performers, failure, dealing with individuals in a competitive context and gender issues.

Tim highlights some potential pitfalls in working with coaches. Some coaches think that the sports psychologist can wave a "magic wand" and everything will be well. Also, sports psychologists are viewed by some coaches as a jargon-wielding, interfering waste of space. The regularity of contact can also be a major issue, and if the contact with the performer is intermittent there is a need to ensure that the coach understands and carries out what the sports psychologist has implemented. However, there is a whole range of positives of working with and through coaches. Tim finds it satisfying enhancing the effectiveness of the performer and the coach, and working in whole range of different contexts and scenarios, which helps him re-assess his working methods at all times. Another positive is the symbiotic learning experience and the expertise that is shared between the performer, coach and sports psychologist, particularly in sports that he is not familiar with.

CONFIDENCE AND CONFIDENCE ENHANCEMENT STRATEGIES

Self-confidence can be a major issue in sports performance, and the smallest thing can have an impact on a performer's self-confidence. Self-confidence is an individual's belief in their ability, and a high level of belief can be critical in whether the performer achieves his or her goals in sport. An example of a high level of belief and goal achievement in sport was seen during a post-match interview with the British Olympic middleweight gold medallist James DeGale during the 2008 Beijing Olympic Games. He acknowledged that after getting through to the quarter finals he knew he would win the gold medal for himself and Great Britain, and he was supremely confident in achieving this goal.

A further example of a confident performer (a subjectively observed assessment) is Manchester United's Cristiano Ronaldo, who during the 2007–8 English soccer season was scoring goals freely for his club. He was always trying new skills, taking shots at goal from a range of angles and distances, and he was always the first one to step up to take a penalty. Generally, confident performers will not be afraid to try anything, while players lacking in confidence avoid responsibility and are afraid of trying things because they feel they will fail.

There are many reasons why a performer may lack self-confidence, such as having far too high expectations of one's ability, which leads to the setting of unrealistic goals. The consequences of not achieving these goals could be loss of concentration and the creeping in of self-doubt, which could subsequently manifest as anxiety and uncertainty of purpose (Martens, 1987).

A range of theories attempts to explain the notion of self-confidence: Harter's (1978) achievement motivation theory suggests that confidence is grounded in an athlete's feelings of competence; Vealey's (1986) sport-specific model of sport confidence suggests that sport confidence concerns the athlete's convictions regarding their competency to achieve sporting success; Nicholls (1984) argues that self-confidence is based on an individual's perceived ability; and Bandura's (1986) theory of self-efficacy refers to an individual's confidence in their competency to achieve a set task (Cox, 1998), which is a crucial element in sport performance.

Bandura's theory argues that self-efficacy is enhanced by four factors: successful performance, vicarious experiences, verbal persuasion and emotional arousal (Cox, 1998). The more success the performer has the more self-confident and self-efficacious they will feel. In the case of Cristiano Ronaldo he possibly feels that the more goals he scores the more he can continue to score. However, Bandura acknowledges that while success can raise expectations for future success, failure can lower them (Cox, 1998), which of course would impact upon self-confidence. Reminders of successful past performance accomplishments can be a powerful tool to engage the performer with. Sports psychologists use reminder sheets listing the good performances achieved as a tool that the performer can carry around with them or put up on their fridge, which is a strategy that the coach can also easily implement and integrate into their practice schedules.

Vicarious experience involves the performer viewing the successful performance of others at a similar level of ability and the coach can develop this by showing the performer videos of other performers who are successful and by providing positive reports on the performer. A third way of developing self-efficacy and self-confidence is by using verbal persuasion; by constructing feedback effectively, the coach can show that they and others have confidence in the performer's abilities. A common technique that sports psychologists use is "self-talk", which is where the performer convinces themselves that they will achieve success. Other persuasive techniques that can be used are acting confident, affirming the positive aspects of performance, team statement exercises and mental imagery (Feltz and Lirgg, 2001). Again, these strategies can be easily implemented and integrated into coaching practice by the coach.

Bartlett et al. (2006, p. 1180) suggest "that self-confidence can influence an athlete's interpretation of emotional arousal", Bandura's fourth factor. For example, sweating and increased heart rate can be perceived by the athlete as a negative aspect of performance preparation, therefore affecting self-confidence. The performer should be persuaded that these responses should be viewed as positive, as it is the body effectively preparing for performance.

The overriding message that should be taken from Bandura's theory is that the coach plays a crucial part in maximizing their performer's levels of self-confidence. The coach should create an environment in training that allows for success, which means setting realistic goals, focusing on the positives and not the negatives of performance, and understanding that the performer can only control the controllables and not the uncontrollables.

CONCENTRATION

Having the ability to concentrate or pay attention for long periods of time on a day-to-day task is difficult. Sport requires the performer to concentrate for long periods of time in a dynamic and constantly changing environment. In some sports the performer is able to get away with drifting in and out of paying attention for small periods of time, such as the golfer walking between holes, and then having to refocus to take a shot on the putting green. Some performers are easily distracted from the task that they should be attending to and find it difficult to refocus. Distractions can be errors in performance, the weather, an opponent, tiredness, or the coach shouting instructions or even negative thoughts entering the mind.

Different sports have different attentional demands, and sports that require prolonged bouts of concentration include, for example the marathon, badminton and tennis. Sports that require intermittent short bursts of concentration include archery, golf, long jump, high jump, pole vault and javelin. Intense levels of concentration are required in sports such as sprinting, surfing and snow-boarding, and sports such as free rock climbing or high diving require a high degree of concentration because the potential for injury if the performer were to be distracted is high. The trouble with not concentrating and not paying attention in sport is that environmental cues are missed. These cues could be relevant and should be attended to, and a performer's ability to attend to relevant cues during competition is known as "attentional focus" (Martens, 1987).

In sport and indeed in general day-to-day activities the individual has the ability to either narrow or broaden their attentional focus and this will depend on the environment and situation they find themselves in (Cox, 1998). For example, the snooker or pool player must be able to broaden his or her attentional focus when stepping up to the snooker table to consider their options for potting a ball, and then narrow their attention as they start cueing to take a shot.

It is suggested by Nideffer (1976) that individuals possess a somewhat permanently fixed attentional style. This could cause problems if the style possessed by the performer does not match that of the situation – the potential for less than successful performance then exists because they would not be able to focus on what are relevant or irrelevant cues in the sports environment. Nideffer developed the Test of Attentional and Interpersonal Style (TAIS) to assess the strengths and weaknesses of an individual's attentional style, which is categorized as broad-internal, broad external, narrow-internal or narrow-external (Nideffer, 1976). It is suggested that different sports require a different attentional focus in different situations (Weinberg and Gould, 2006).

A range of strategies exists that can help the performer refocus, and they can easily be implemented in training as well as competition. Use of triggers, such as slapping a thigh, clicking the fingers or rotating a racket in the hand three times before serving are time honoured strategies that can be used to enable the performer to regain their focus on the task in hand. Trigger or cue words can also be used to regain attentional focus and concentrate. The words used can be anything from "set", "execute", "stop shot", and are unique to the individual performer.

This author has used cue words for field hockey players on a regular basis. In field hockey when a short corner is given, in order to enable the short corner injector to refocus after the mêlée in the circle that resulted in the short corner, three cue words are provided. These cue words are "set" (the injector breathing out and setting themselves for skill execution), "smooth" (executing the skill in a smooth motion) and "straight" (ensuring that the ball delivery is straight to the top of the circle). Another strategy that is available to the coach and is of special importance prior to competition is either a pre-competition or pre-event routine (these will be looked at in more detail later on in this chapter).

MOTIVATION AND DEVELOPMENT OF A MOTIVATIONAL CLIMATE

The coach should be an excellent motivator. Although a range of strategies are used to motivate performers, the coach should have a good understanding of how and why these strategies work, and how to engineer a successful motivational climate in training and competition. What motivates a performer to come to training in the depths of winter? What motivates a performer to seek perfection in skill execution? What of the gifted performer who for no reason gives up playing a sport; what is their motivation for doing this?

Motivation can be defined as "the direction and intensity of one's effort" (Sage, 1977 cited in Weinberg and Gould, 2006, p. 52). The direction equates to the choice of activity or the goals being aspired to and the intensity equates to the effort and persistence that is allocated to the task. There are two basic types of motivation, intrinsic and extrinsic. Being intrinsically motivated is doing the activity for its own sake and being extrinsically motivated is doing the activity for some form of reward or praise (Cox, 1998, 2007; Horn, 1992; McMorris and Hale, 2006). Intrinsically motivated performers tend to:

- Enjoy their sport more, are self-confident and have higher levels of self-esteem.
- Adhere to training programmes longer.
- Concentrate better and are task driven.
- Be less anxious and have more peak performances.

(Vallerand, 2001)

Generally, the motivational patterns of those performers who are extrinsically motivated are completely opposite to motivational patterns of those who are intrinsically motivated. Detling (2008) argues that there are three primary motivation killers: perfectionism, expectations and comparisons. Considering these, the coach should make efforts to educate those performers who are always striving for perfectionism that practice makes *permanent*, not perfect. They should try and reduce the too high expectations of performers to a more realistic level, and help the performer to understand that they are their own person, and making comparisons is illogical because they can never be the same as someone else. Players define success differently and their definitions are referred to as achievement-goal orientations (Hodge, 2004).

There are two major goal orientations; task or mastery, and outcome or ego orientation. A task oriented performer's success focus is on mastering a task or skill, and an ego oriented performer's success focus is on social comparison, in that they compare their ability against that of others of a similar ability. The coach should aim to create a positive motivational climate in training and competition, and one which fosters a task or mastery goal orientation.

The coach should also structure practices in a way that fosters mutual reciprocation and features goal achievement that is challenging yet attainable for the athletes. The coach should also plan and organize training programmes and keep open communication channels, which will also result in the development of mutual respect between coach and athletes. It is crucial that the coach remains impartial, supportive and consistent when winning or losing, and identifies any obstructions in the coaching process and implements strategies to circumvent them (Weiss, 2004).

ANXIETY AND AROUSAL

Cox (1998) suggests anxiety can be viewed as being either situation-specific or general in nature and divided into two components, state anxiety and trait anxiety. State anxiety is an emotional condition that sees a rise in physiological arousal, and trait anxiety is a personality issue, in which the individual views certain situations as threatening and will respond with a rise in their levels of state anxiety (Spielberger, 1971).

A range of theories attempts to explain the causes of anxiety and the potential effect on performance. There is Hardy and Fazey's (1987) catastrophe theory, which argues that when performers go over the top of an inverted U-curve, performance reduces suddenly rather than gradually. Eysenck and Calvo's (1992) processing efficiency theory predicts that anxiety takes up some of the processing and storage resources of a limited capacity working memory system (the mind), a consequence of which is that elevated levels of anxiety place high demands on the capacity of the working memory system (Hardy *et al.*, 2007). Hardy and co-workers add that a second important prediction of processing efficiency theory is that anxiety can serve a motivational purpose. Martens *et al.*'s (1990) multi-dimensional anxiety theory argues for a cognitive and somatic component each having dissimilar effects on performance and in theory both components can be manipulated independently of one another.

A plethora of questionnaires exists that purport to measure levels of anxiety, and one of the most used and popular is the Competitive Sport Anxiety Inventory-2 (CSAI-2) (Martens et al., 1990 cited in Cox, 1998), which measures anxiety from a multi-dimensional perspective, something many other questionnaires are not able to do. The CSAI-2 is used to determine pre-competition levels of cognitive and somatic anxiety, and also has a directional scale. Cognitive anxiety is described as the mental component of state anxiety and is caused by things such as fear of failure, and somatic anxiety is the physical component of anxiety that manifests itself in responses such as increased heart and breathing rate, and muscle tension (Cox, 1998, 2007; Horn, 2008). Both cognitive and somatic anxiety symptomatic of state anxiety, which is seen as changeable rather than the more stable trait anxiety component. The CSAI-2 also has a directional scale which determines whether the performer perceives what he or she is feeling is either facilitative (good) or debilitative (bad).

Understanding the "time to event" framework is also crucial for the coach, because those performers who suffer from the effects of anxiety will probably go through a process that see cognitive anxiety levels elevated but stable as competition approaches, and somatic anxiety levels staying low. At around a day prior to competition somatic anxiety levels will rise, and on starting competition both cognitive and somatic anxiety will decrease (Hardy and Parfitt, 1991; Martens et al., 1990). This is a general perspective on the "time to event" framework and there will obviously be individual differences in performer's anxiety states over time.

Having a good understanding of the time to event framework can help the coach understand how different performers will respond in different ways prior to competition. Some performers who are naturally bubbly and enthusiastic can become quiet and slightly withdrawn, and visit the toilet more often prior to competition, while others who are normally quiet may become more talkative. These are some of the outward signs of a change in behaviour prior to competition, and the longer the coach has worked with their performers the greater will be their understanding of how each performer deals with the upcoming challenge of competition.

Cognitive anxiety reduction strategies such as reducing the importance of competition, implementing an effective goal setting programme and the use of pre-performance routines (Martens, 1987), together with somatic anxiety intervention strategies such as breathing, parking and relaxation techniques (Bull et al., 1996) are easily implemented and integrated into coaching programmes. However, for the more severe cases of anxiety the coach should recommend that the services of a sports psychologist should be sought.

Anxiety and arousal are used interchangeably to explain how some performers respond to the challenges of training and competition. However, there should be a distinction made between anxiety and arousal. "The state of being anxious as a result of an environmental stimulus is associated with an elevation in arousal" (Cox, 1998, p. 86), and "arousal is the physiological and or the cognitive readiness to act" (McMorris, 2004, p. 242).

Similar to anxiety, a range of theories attempts to explain the arousal performance relationship. These include Yerkes and Dodson's (1908) inverted U theory, which argues for an optimal level of arousal; Hull's (1943) drive theory, which argues that arousal increases in a linear fashion; Easterbrook's (1959) cue utilization theory, which argues that the individual utilizes either relevant or irrelevant cues in the environment; and Kahneman's (1973) allocatable resources theory, which argues that the organism allocates resources to the task in hand and performance on one or more tasks suffers when the resource demands of the tasks exceed available supply (Szalma and Hancock, 2009).

McMorris and Hale (2006) suggest that changes in arousal are caused by positive or negative emotions, and anxiety is one of the negative emotions that causes increases in arousal. However, arousal can be used positively. In some sports such as the shot put, weightlifting and rugby, elevated levels of arousal are required to energize the mind and body in order to prepare for performance. Conversely, low levels of arousal are required for sports such as archery and snooker in which calm and controlled skill execution is required.

Unfortunately, some sports performers get over-aroused and get a "rush of blood to the head", or the "red mist" takes over. Consequences of this include being penalized by a referee for a reckless tackle or injury to themselves or other performers. Other performers can "freeze" or "choke" when they are about to perform, and Nideffer and Sagal (2001) suggest that choking is a common response in the sporting environment when an athlete is under competition stress. The skill of the coach is knowing when the performer is beginning to get over-aroused in competition, or when they are not aroused enough. If the coach is in a sport where substitutions can be made it would probably be prudent to substitute a player who is beginning to get over-aroused, as much to protect the player as others around them.

Arousal reduction strategies are much the same as the somatic anxiety reducers (breathing and relaxation techniques) and soft relaxing music can also be used. If the coach wants to energize the performer, or if the performer wants to energize themselves then either a rousing team or pep talk, or up-beat music (Bull *et al.*, 1996) can be used.

IMAGERY

Humans are able to visualize and produce images in their "mind's eye". In sport, performers are able to re-create vivid images in their mind, for example of that special goal scored or skill or performance that they executed. Coaches of young children often use visual images that represent a skill in an easy to understand language and form, in order for the child to understand the context of the movement. For example, in field hockey quite often the coach, when asking the young performer to get into a knees bent and back straight position to receive the ball in a balanced position, says "Imagine yourself sitting on the toilet". The children are then able to visualize the correct position to be in to receive the ball. Use of imagery in the adult context is no different, and many performers, depending on their learning style, are able to visualize the skill before they execute it.

In essence, imagery can be defined as involving the ability of a performer to "mentally recreate objects, persons, skills, experiences and situations, while not actually physically involved in these situations" (Hodge, 2004, p. 124). Imagery, like physical skills, is a practised skill, and is useful when practising motor skills. However, the performer must ensure that the visual representation they are imagining is an exact replica of the physical skill, otherwise incorrect movement patterns may be mentally practised. Imagery is not to be confused with mental practice.

Mental imagery is regarded as a mental process and mental practice as a particular technique (Murphy and Jowdry, 1992 cited in Cox, 1998). Researchers are not fully sure how the process works, but it is generally thought that imagery provides a mental blueprint of the skill or performance (Sheik and Korn, 1994). More recently, researchers from the University of Birmingham (UK) have reported that neurons first discovered in the brains of monkeys could help us understand why mental imagery is beneficial for athletes (Burns, 2005).

When using imagery, performers should practise in a distraction-free environment, practise systematically and attempt to make the image as vivid as possible (Morris *et al.*, 2005).

Performers should try and re-create as much of the environment they compete in as possible, e.g. the feeling of warmth or coldness, sound and smell.

There are two types of imagery: external and internal. External imagery is when the performer views themselves as if on film, and internal imagery is when the performer actually feels the movement from within their own body (McMorris and Hale, 2006). For example, the baseball pitcher using external imagery would see themselves from a distance throwing an accurate and fast ball. When using internal imagery the baseball pitcher throwing a ball would feel the throwing arm recoil, the pivoting on one leg, rotation of the trunk, transfer of weight and extension of the throwing arm to release the ball.

What is also important for both external and internal imagery is to imagine not only performance, but also the outcome. So, taking the baseball pitcher as an example again, seeing and hearing the ball go through the air and making a smacking sound as it lands in the catcher's gloves should also form part of the imagery process. A good example of a top sports performer using imagery is England rugby player Jonny Wilkinson. He claims that his hand-clasping helps him blot out the outside world as he imagines a wire connected between the ball and the space between the posts. All he then has to do is kick the ball such that it follows the wire. "Doris" forms another component of Wilkinson's mental training. This involves him aiming to kick the ball into the lap of Doris, an imaginary woman who sits in a particular seat holding an ice cream. The aim is to knock the ice cream out of her hands (Wertperch, 2008).

At the 2004 Athens Olympics, Herste Cloete, the South African high jumper, went through an intricate pre-performance routine prior to each jump, which involved using imagery. She closed her eyes and went through a series of fine finger and hand movements that represented her run-up, take-off, flight over the high jump bar and landing.

Many theories attempt to explain how and why imagery works, and two of the main ones are Sackett's (1934) symbolic learning theory and Carpenter's (1984 cited in Plessinger, 2008) psychoneuromuscular theory. Psychoneuromuscular theory suggests that vivid, imagined events produce neuromuscular responses similar to those of an actual experience. It seems that the images in the brain actually cause muscular contractions so small that no movement actually takes place, but the pathway is utilized. The second main theory is symbolic learning theory. This theory suggests that imagery develops a coding system of movement patterns, thereby creating a mental blueprint in the central nervous system.

PRE-PERFORMANCE ROUTINES

The use of ritualistic and superstitious behaviours is endemic in sport (Bleak and Frederick, 1998). Superstitious behaviours can come in the form of the use of lucky charms, pre- and post-game activity or the wearing of specific clothing (Burhmann et al., 1982). These rituals or routines can begin days before the start of an event, right up to the point of the starting whistle or starting gun. In the day leading up to competition a typical routine might be for a team sports player to get up at a specific time, have the same breakfast at the same time and go through a routine of packing their kit in a specific order. They might leave the house at an exact time and follow the same route to the venue. When they are changing into their sports kit, they might put their kit on in a certain way (e.g. left sock first) and have a "lucky" piece of kit that they wear. When going into the arena, they might go out in a specific place in the team, and go through a final routine before the competition starts.

A pre-performance routine is a sequence of events that an athlete systematically carries out prior to performance (Moran, 1996) and vary from sport to sport and from skill to skill.

Pre-performance routines are more specific than ritualistic and superstitious behaviours and are conducted immediately prior to performance. Many sports men and women consciously (or indeed unconsciously) go through a pre-performance routine. Many tennis players bounce around on their feet prior to receiving a serve, or bounce the ball a number of times prior to serving. Lidor and Singer (2000, p. 35) suggest performers use pre-performance routines "to facilitate learning and performance and give performers control over their motor, emotional, and cognitive behaviours".

Furthermore, many performers use pre-competition routines as a psychological preparation tool for the challenge of training and competition (Martens, 1987). To be effective, pre-performance routines must be practised, the length of the routine must be consistent and execution of the routine must occur at the same time prior to the execution of the skill (Cox, 1998).

GOAL SETTING

In 1979 Locke and Latham published a landmark paper that presented their research on the self-regulation and motivation of logging industry workers in the USA. Their findings suggested that when individuals are able to set their own goals and they are provided with the support and resources they need to achieve those goals, productivity increases (Smith-Nash, 2005). Goal setting is now popular in sport, and a solid base of evidence suggests that goal setting influences behaviour and helps increase motivation and self-confidence while reducing anxiety and social conflict (Weinberg and Gould, 2006).

Goal setting can be defined as "attaining a standard of proficiency on a task, usually within a specified period of time" (Locke and Latham, 1985, p. 705) or setting an objective, having an aim or attaining a level of performance (Weinberg and Gould, 1999). Two theoretical views are put forward to explain why goal setting works. The mechanistic view (Locke and Latham, 1985), which is not sport-specific, suggests that goal setting focuses attention, enhances effort, increases persistence and encourages the individual to think about and develop a range of different perspectives. The cognitive view, which is more sport-specific, suggests that goal setting elevates self-motivation, self-confidence, pleasure in participating in the sport and that it can also reduce anxiety (Burton, 1989).

Different types of goals exist, such as dream goals, which may be winning an Olympic gold medal; outcome goals, such as winning a competition or race; performance goals, which are numeric and include, for example, beating a personal best; and process goals, such as improving techniques or skills (Weinberg and Gould, 1999), and all have their strengths and weaknesses. Setting specific, difficult yet attainable process goals has been associated with higher motivation and sport performance (Locke and Latham, 1990; Zimmerman and Kitsantas, 1996) and this can be easily done by the coach in training. Research has found, however, that the setting of multiple goals can also be effective (Filby *et al.*, 1999). Goals also need to be considered from a short-, medium- and long-term perspective. Goals should be challenging but not so difficult that they are unattainable and not so easy that they are easily attainable.

Martens (1987) recommends the "staircase" approach to goal setting, whereby the immediate goal is set only slightly above the previous performance average. A series of steps are then planned, each being progressively more difficult, to achieve the final goal. Unfortunately, common mistakes occur when goals are set, and although they are easy to administer, they are often not implemented effectively. Goal setting can be time consuming, and although goals are implemented with good intentions at the start of a season, they can fall by the wayside.

Coaches not fully understanding the mechanics and processes of goal setting sometimes only set outcome goals (e.g. win the league) which the performer is not in control of, or they set too many goals and the performer does not participate in the process. The SMARTER mnemonic should be incorporated into the goal setting programme, which is expanded as follows:

S – Specific. Goals should be specific. "I want to decrease my 50 m butterfly stroke swim time".

M – Measurable. The goal should be quantifiable. "I want to decrease my 50 m butterfly stroke swim time by one second".

A – Agreed. The goals should be agreed by the performer and coach.

R – Realistic. The goal should be challenging and not difficult. It should not be too easy, which might reduce the performer's motivation.

T – Time phased. The goal should be achieved by the agreed date.

E – Exciting. The goal needs to be exciting to motivate the performer.

R – Recorded. The goal should be written down to increase the performer's commitment to the goal, and to help evaluate progress.

(Adapted from Cox, 1998; Crisfield *et al.*, 2003; Martens, 1987)

SUMMARY

Psychologists function in a range of sub-disciplines including educational, clinical, counselling, research and applied; and sports psychologists fall into three main categories of educational, research or applied. Sports psychology is a science in which social psychology principles are applied in a sport or exercise setting, and are often applied to enhance sport and exercise performance (Cox, 1998, p. 4). The role and function of the sports psychologist in the USA has been regulated and professionalized for many years and organizations in the UK such as the British Psychological Society (BPS) and British Association of Sport and Exercise Sciences (BASES) have and are also further developing processes in which those wishing to become a sports psychologist have to be accredited and certified competent to practice.

Coaches who are successful integrate a range of psychological strategies into their technical, tactical and fitness programmes, and are usually good 'man' managers. It is crucial that the coach understands that the sports psychologist should be utilized in a supporting role, and is not there to undermine the coach, as it is the coach who has the ultimate responsibility of performance outcomes. However, if the coach requires the services of a sports psychologist they should contact BASES or the BPS who will be able to provide details of accredited practitioners.

The coach or sports psychologist is able to implement mental skills training into the overall training programme, such as confidence enhancement, concentration strategies, motivation, anxiety reduction, imagery, pre-performance routines and a goal setting programme.

SEMINAR OR DISCUSSION QUESTIONS

1. Describe how a coach could develop a positive motivational climate for their performers.
2. Explain the differences between types of goals.

KEY TERMS AND DEFINITIONS

- Arousal – the physiological and/or cognitive readiness to act.
- Concentration – having the ability to attend to cues in the environment for prolonged periods of time.
- Extrinsic motivation – doing the activity for reward of praise.
- Goal – an objective, aim of some action or level of performance.
- Imagery – ability to mentally re-create objects, persons, skills, experiences and situations while not physically being involved in these situations.
- Intrinsic motivation – doing the activity for its own sake.
- Motivation – the direction and intensity of one's effort.
- Pre-performance routine – a sequence of task-relevant thoughts and actions which an athlete systematically engages in prior to his or her performance of a specific sport skill.
- Self-confidence – an individual's belief in their ability.
- Sports psychology – a science in which the principles of psychology are applied in the sport and exercise setting.
- State of anxiety – an emotional state that sees an elevation in physiological arousal.
- Trait anxiety – a personality variable.

WEB LINKS

Athletic Insight – www.athleticinsight.com
British Association of Sport and Exercise Sciences (BASES) – www.bases.org.uk
British Psychological Society (BPS) Division of Sport and Exercise Psychology – www.bps.org.uk
Mental strength – www.mentalstrength.com
Mind Tools – www.mindtools.com

FURTHER READING

Bull, S. J., Albinson, J. G. and Shambrook, J. (1996). *The Mental Game Plan: Getting Psyched for Sport*. Sports Dynamics, Eastbourne.
Cox, R. H. (1998). *Sport Psychology: Concepts and Applications* (4th edn). McGraw-Hill, New York.
Cox, R. H. (2007). *Sport Psychology: Concepts and Applications* (6th edn). McGraw-Hill, New York.
Hardy, L. and Parfitt, G. (1991). A Catastrophe Model of Anxiety and Performance. *British Journal of Psychology*, 82, 163–78.
Hodge, K. (2004). *The Complete Guide to Sport Motivation*. A & C Black, London.

Horn, T. S. (1992). *Advances in Sport Psychology* (1st edn). Human Kinetics, Champaign, IL.
Horn, T. S. (2008). *Advances in Sport Psychology* (3rd edn). Human Kinetics, Champaign, IL.
Jarvis, M. (2006). *Sports Psychology: A Student's Handbook*. Routledge, London.
Martens, R. (1987). *The Coaches Guide to Sports Psychology*. Human Kinetics, Champaign, IL.
Moran, A. P. (2003). *Sport and Exercise Psychology: A Critical Introduction*. Routledge, London.

Chapter 14

Skill acquisition and the role of the coach

CHAPTER OBJECTIVES

- Differentiate between skill and ability.
- Explain the process of learning.
- Explain the role of memory.
- Explain selective attention.
- Explain decision making.
- Explain anticipation.
- Explain reaction time.
- Explain feedback.
- Identify and describe the different types of practice.

SKILL AND ABILITY

"Skill can be defined as the ability to bring about pre-determined results with maximum certainty often with the minimum outlay of time, energy or both" (Knapp, 1963, p. 4). Davis *et al.* (1995, p. 231) suggest that skill has an "end result, which means it is goal directed". All sporting movement is skilled, and the main differences between the novice and skilled performer are: skilled performers are more consistent in repeating performance; skilled performers execute skills with efficient use of energy and in a coordinated manner; and skilled performers are more practised in their sport. Schmidt (1991) suggests there are three critical elements to almost any skill: perceiving the relevant environmental features, deciding what to do and where and when to do it, and organizing the muscles to generate movements. Ericsson and Smith (1991) suggest that different types of skill exist, which include:

- Cognitive skills – involve thought and problem solving such as the boxing judge calculating the points scored in a 3 x 3 minute round amateur contest.
- Fundamental motor skills – basic skills, such as the young child running, jumping, catching, kicking and throwing while at play.
- Motor skills – movements such as Joe DiMaggio hitting a baseball with his baseball bat.
- Perceptual motor skills – skills that allow the performer to make sense of an approaching

stimulus and execute movement, such as the badminton player Nathan Robertson assessing the flight of the shuttlecock and moving to impact the shuttlecock with his badminton racket.

■ Perceptual skills – skills that help the performer make sense of the environment and make a decision based on the information in the environment. For example, the tennis player assessing the ball flight of a service as it is coming over the net, and making a decision as to what shot to employ for the return.

Presenting different skills on a continuum, within their respective classifications, will enable the coach to understand the nature of individual skills and teach them effectively. Table 14.1 highlights how skills are classified, with practical examples of each.

The word "ability" is used in psychology to describe existing foundation actions that underlie skilled performance (McMorris, 2004). Abilities are thought of as being largely genetic and something that the individual is born with (Honeybourne, 2006). Having ability, whether it is in music, languages, mathematics or sport, provides the individual with the basis from which to learn skills and Schmidt (1991) argues that ability is essentially unchanged by practice or experience. There is debate as to whether an individual has groups of abilities or specific ones.

During the 1950s and 1960s, Henry and Fleishman investigated the abilities of hundreds of students and military personnel. While both researchers concluded that there was no such thing as general motor ability, Fleishman believed that individuals display groups of abilities and Henry argued for specific and unique abilities (McMorris 2004). For example, Fleishman would argue that static, dynamic and explosive strength would be clustered (grouped) together as components of strength while Henry would argue that they were each unique abilities. While disagreement persists over whether an individual possesses specific or groups of abilities, Jarvis has recently put forward the concept of "superability", which has "some effect on but does not directly determine specific motor abilities" (Jarvis, 1999, p. 117).

In broad terms, it has been shown that when athletes are tested they exhibit high scores in a range of different abilities. Anecdotally, it would seem that some individuals have a natural ability to perform a multitude of sports with ease, and the UK Sport Talent Transfer

Table 14.1 Skill classification continua

Fine motor skills	Gross motor skills	
Small muscle action (Dart throwing)	Large muscle action (Weightlifting)	
Open skills	Closed skills	
Changeable environment (Open play in rugby, soccer, field hockey)	Stable environment (Basketball free throw shot)	
Externally paced	Self-paced	
Environment determines start of the skill (Windsurfing)	Performer determines the start (Gymnastics – asymmetric bars)	
Continuous	Serial	Discrete
Unclear beginning and end of cycle (Running)	Several discrete tasks joined in quick succession (Triple jump)	Clear beginning and end (Squash serve)

programme has identified performers with natural talent in one sport that can be utilized in another. For example, Rebecca Romero, the 2004 Olympic rowing silver medallist, switched to track cycling and won the National Championships less than a year later. She then went on to win silver in her first international World Cup event. Arguably, it could be that rowing and cycling have a cluster of abilities that are unique to those sports. However, although many individuals appear to be good in a range of sports and may have a good general motor ability, research evidence is not able to fully support this claim (McMorris, 2004).

LEARNING

Learning is behaviour development or the acquiring of information that is not genetically determined or a result of previous experience (Allaby, 1999). The capability to learn is essential to human existence (Schmidt and Wrisberg, 2000) and the coach is in a unique position to provide the performer with effective learning experiences. Understanding how the performer learns is critical because the coach can then structure practice and provide feedback in order to optimize performance. Some performers have a unique capability to assimilate information and learn quickly while others need more guidance, and arguably one of the main factors that the coach needs to consider is the performer's individual learning style, which is outlined in Chapter 5.

Two competing schools of thought have emerged that attempt to explain how we learn. There are the information processing theorists who believe that learning is all to do with memory; and the ecological psychologists who believe that memory has no role in learning and all that we need to do to achieve the task is to search for cues (affordances) in the environment (McMorris, 2004). Both schools have appeal, and coaching is conducted using both perspectives.

When coaching from an information processing approach, the coach goes through a mechanistic process which is instructional in nature, providing coaching points, a demonstration, letting the performer practice and giving feedback and error correction.

When delivering from an ecological perspective the coach just provides the basic task and by using guided discovery lets the performer explore the environment through trial and error to work out which is the best way to achieve the task. A one-year-old child who picks up a ball for the first time has not been coached to throw the ball, but they explore the action of picking up the ball, what it feels like, how to throw it, how it bounces, where it lands and then how to crawl or run after it. Basically, they are exploring the environment. A range of theories attempts to explain how performers learn, two of which have been selected for this section (for further information on learning theories see the suggested further reading at the end of this chapter).

Fitts and Posner (1967) suggest that skill is learned in three stages, which they describe as the cognitive, associative and autonomous phases. In the cognitive phase the athlete forms a mental picture, identifying and developing the component parts of the skill. In the associative phase the athlete will physically link the component parts together, and feedback and practice is required to reinforce learning in order to perfect the skills. In the autonomous phase the athlete continues to develop and practise the learned skill so that it becomes automatic, involving little or no conscious thought or attention while performing the skill.

Vygotsky (1978) suggests that we learn through a process of "conceptual behavioural modelling". An example of this would be the coach explaining what they are thinking and doing as they model the skill. The performer identifies the relevant behaviours (techniques) required and then develops a mental blueprint of the technique(s). The performer then attempts to reproduce those behaviours (techniques) with the coach observing, monitoring, analysing and providing error correction (feedback), which is, in essence, coaching. It is "coaching that provides assistance at the most critical level, the skill level just beyond what the learner could accomplish themself" (Edmondson, 2005, p. 21). Vygotsky refers to this as the "zone of proximal development" and believes that promoting skill/technique development in this zone leads to accelerated learning.

Learning also comes in two guises: implicit and explicit learning. Explicit learning is learning after being given instructions, which is a predominant feature of coaching. Implicit learning is learning at a subconscious level: Magill (1993) and Masters (2000 cited in McMorris, 2004) have shown that exposure to a skill, even if the performer is not consciously paying attention to it, can result in learning of at least as good a value as when it is learnt explicitly. Raab (2003) has suggested that in low complexity task situations implicit learners (learning at a sub-conscious level) perform better than explicit learners (learning through instruction), and in high complexity task situations the opposite is true.

MEMORY

Eysenck and Keane (2005) suggest that memory can be represented as a multi-store system. This multi-store system is inclusive of the sensory store (SS), which holds information for around 250 milliseconds; short-term memory (STM) which holds information for around 30 seconds; and long-term memory (LTM) which is capable of holding information for long periods of time (Schmidt and Wrisberg, 2000). All the information that passes through the SS does not reach consciousness because individuals are only able to process a limited amount of information from the vast amount of information that they are exposed to. Therefore, a selective attention mechanism selects some sensory information in the SS for further processing and the remainder of the information in the SS is lost and then replaced by more recent sensory information (Schmidt, 1991).

Focusing of attention lengthens the period during which the information is stored in the STM (Davis et al., 1995), therefore when the coach is delivering a new skill to a new learner it is critical that they provide an accurate demonstration coupled with concise and accurate verbal cues to support the demonstration. When initially performing the skill the performer, through the process of selective attention, will use the STM to store the new information learned and transfer it to the LTM. To achieve this they will have to rehearse (practise) the skill straightaway in order to remember the key coaching points and what the demonstration looked like. The main issue with transferring information from the STM to the LTM is that the STM has to recall from the LTM a past experience of the particular skill being learnt. If that past experience does not exist, then the new skill has to be reinforced through feedback, error correction and continued practice in order for the performer to commit the newly learned skill to their LTM.

A further issue exists in terms of the capacity of the STM. In 1956 George Armitage Miller, an American psychologist, published a seminal research paper suggesting that 7 + 2 was the magic number that characterized people's memory performance on random lists of letters, words, numbers or almost any kind of meaningful familiar item (McMorris, 2004; Schmidt, 1991; Schmidt and Wrisberg, 2000). This has implications for the coach when coaching children, because Miller also suggested that this magic number of seven was much lower in children (McMorris, 2004). However, more recently Cowan (2001) has proposed that working memory (STM) has a capacity of about four "chunks" in young adults (and less in children and old adults). Therefore, the coach must consider how much information and feedback they are providing the performer, especially in the earlier stages of learning.

There are many reasons why we forget things. Sometimes information never reaches the LTM, other times the information gets there but is lost. Other reasons include memory deterioration, and on top of this it is possible that we are physiologically pre-programmed to erase data that is no longer relevant to us after a period of time (Heffner, 2001). Whether this can be applied in the sporting context is open to debate. For example, many people learn to ride a bicycle when they are very young, then as they get older and pass their driving test the car becomes the easier option. However, even after many years of not using a bicycle many people are able to easily get onto a bicycle (albeit a bit unsure at first) and execute the skill of cycling with ease.

SELECTIVE ATTENTION

In sport the performer is exposed to an inordinate amount of information, of which only a certain amount is relevant and can be processed at one time. Therefore, the performer needs a have a mechanism by which they can cognitively sift through this information, sifting what is relevant from what is irrelevant, and this is called selective attention.

Filter models, which seek to explain the process of selective attention, are used as a theoretical underpinning. Broadbent (1958 cited in McMorris, 2004) contends that while all information enters the STM, we only attend to selected stimuli (signals, patterns). Norman (1969, cited in McMorris 2004) suggests that the key factor in attending to relevant cues is "pertinence", which means that the importance of the stimulus will determine whether we attend to it or not. More recently, Treisman (1998) has proposed what she calls the feature binding model. Treisman contends that information presented is bound together as a feature within the environmental display. These features have different parts, and Triesman argues that individuals select one object for binding at a time, so that the parts of the irrelevant objects do not compete in the binding process.

Being able to read an opponent effectively comes with experience of knowing what signals or cues to look for, and good coaching (Robinson, 2006c). In fast ball sports it is crucial that the performer recognizes movement patterns or signals that are being displayed by their opponent(s) and attends to the relevant cues so that they can make the correct response.

For example, cricket batsmen had to attempt to read Shane Warne's or Jason Gillespie's bowling actions in order to execute the correct batting response. International batsmen through experience know what particular patterns or signals are presented by the bowler, such as speed of approach, angle and orientation of hips and shoulders, position of arm, elbow and hand, and of course the release of the ball and ball flight, which is all relevant information that needs attending to in order to execute the right response. Within the visual field of the batsman there is also a lot of irrelevant information, such as the noise of the crowd and position of the umpire, that does not need attending to. If the batsman was trying to process all the information that was available around them, then potentially the relevant cues of the bowling action would be missed, resulting in an incorrect response being executed, which could result in being bowled out.

The coach can engineer coaching sessions by putting the performer in "what if" situations where the performer is coached to recognize which information is relevant and which irrelevant. For example, the soccer coach working with a defender on defending skills could manipulate different patterns of movement presented by an attacker, e.g. the Cruyff turn and cutting in with the left or right foot, and at the same time ask the defender a question,

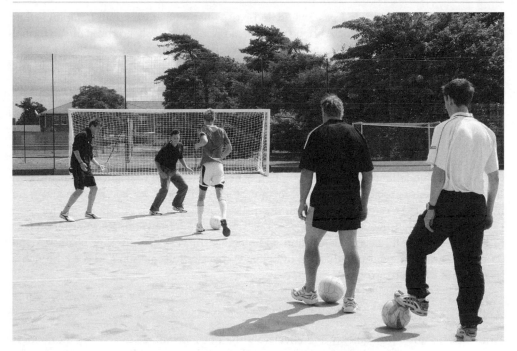

Photo 14.1 A coach pointing out relevant cues for the defender to attend to.

such as "What if the attacker's body was in that position, which way would they turn?" This strategy can be used to enable the defender to build up a visual representation of the relevant signals and patterns that are being provided, in order for them to make the right response. The coach would then put this into a game context situation, where irrelevant as well as relevant cues would exist, and constantly expose the defender to practice schedules that would provide realistic situations in which they would have to filter out the relevant cues that need attending to.

DECISION MAKING

There are some performers who are able to execute a skill, such as passing in soccer, netball, basketball and rugby, seemingly effortlessly and accurately. They are able to pick out a pass to a team member with time and space to spare, and are game aware, knowing what space to move into. There are also players who are a source of frustration to coaches, who after going through a series of tactical situations in training are unable during competition to make the correct decision.

Decision making is in part associated with the ability to scan the visual field effectively (Knudson and Kluka, 1997) to learn what is relevant or irrelevant (selective attention) and is in part associated with our perceptual abilities, i.e. the performer tries to make sense of the information that is presented to them. In sport, visual attention is required to detect, recognize, recall and select stimuli for higher level processing when a decision has to be made and carried out in the form of a motor response (Starkes and Ericsson, 2003).

Simply put, decision making is knowing what to do, when to do it and how to do it. For example, on receiving the ball the field hockey player could be considering decisions, such as do I still carry the ball? do I pass? when do I pass? what type of pass shall I employ? what shall I do when I have passed? Although players do not consciously go through the formal process of asking themselves the questions, past experience, which is held in the LTM, and the scanning of the visual field (that is providing their head is up) will play a part in the decision they make.

Schmidt (1975) proposed schema theory in an effort to explain how we make decisions. He suggested that we do not try to recall specific and precise past situations (from LTM), but instead recall a generalized set of rules or schemas of what decision to make in a situation. These schemas "allow us to make an accurate decision regardless of differences between the present situation and past experience" (McMorris, 2004, p. 178).

Cognitive modelling and sequential sampling models – an area of science that deals with simulating human problem solving and mental processes using a computerized model – are now being adapted to attempt to explain the decision making process in sport, and Johnson (2006) suggests that the use of cognitive models in sport offers advantages in other aspects of behaviour as well, such as perception and memory. In very broad terms, cognitive and sequential modelling suggests that the individual processes information and goes through a sequence of events to arrive at a decision.

ANTICIPATION

Being able to anticipate quickly and effectively is a huge advantage in sports performance, and allows the performer to make a decision and respond to it quickly. Anticipation can be simply defined as the ability to have an expectation of, or to predict, upcoming events in the visual field. McMorris (2004) suggests that anticipation explains how we are able to execute actions, such as catching, hitting a shuttlecock or kicking a ball, that require a degree of interception.

Performers are able to intercept moving objects that are moving at incredible speeds. The field hockey player is able to receive a pass that is moving at around 130 km/h (80 mph) and professional tennis players are able to get into position to return a Roger Federer serve at around 200 km/h (125 mph). More important than the speed of Federer's serve is his ability to produce accurate serves at different angles and bounces using the same serving motion (Zaheen, 2008), which causes more anticipatory problems for his opponent.

Poulton (1957) describes interceptive actions as "coincidence anticipation", and divides this into "effector anticipation", which is the performer's ability to make a decision on how long it will take to move their body, and "receptor anticipation", which is the performer's ability to make a decision on how long it will take an event to occur. For example, the field hockey goal keeper needs to anticipate how long it will take the ball to come into range so the save can be made (receptor anticipation) and how long it will take them to get their body into position to make the save (effector anticipation).

Poulton calls the ability to predict upcoming events "perceptual anticipation" and plays a significant role in the performer being able to predict upcoming events with limited available information (Poulton, 1950). Perceptual anticipation integrates three other types of anticipation: spatial, event and temporal anticipation (McMorris, 2004; Schmidt, 1991; Schmidt and Wrisberg, 2000). Spatial anticipation refers to *where* a performer thinks an action will happen, e.g. the field hockey defender moving to a position to close down space that he or she thinks will be utilized by an opposition forward. Event anticipation is predicting *what* will happen, e.g. the field hockey defender predicting that a forward will attack the open space. Temporal anticipation is predicting *when* an event will occur, e.g. the field hockey defender anticipating the moment a forward will decide to move into the open space.

There is a strong advantage in knowing when some events will happen but it is probably more important for performers to be able to anticipate what is going to happen in order for them to organize their movements in advance (Schmidt, 1991; Schmidt and Wrisberg, 2000). Researchers have investigated the differences between novice and expert performers, and although there may be anecdotal evidence to suggest that "experts possess superior visual systems than novices", it seems that anticipation in sport is "due to enhanced computational sophistication and improved strategic processing of sport-specific information rather than to differences in visual abilities" (Williams, 2002, p. 417).

REACTION TIME

Reaction time is the speed at which we make decisions, and being able to respond quicker than your opponent in, for example, the 100 metres is an obvious advantage. Usain Bolt and Oscar Pistorius, in the 2008 Beijing Olympics and Paralympic Games respectively, were both slow starters out of the blocks in their 100 m finals but were able to increase their acceleration to win a gold medal, which raises an interesting question: If they were able to react quicker on the start, how much quicker would their times have been? Responding to a stimulus, e.g. the starting gun in a sprint race, is a complex affair, and to understand how a performer initiates a reaction, differentiation must be made between reaction, response and movement times.

Reaction time is the time from the introduction of the stimulus to the beginning of the response; response time is the time from the introduction of the stimulus to the end of the response; and movement time is the time from the beginning of the response to the end of the response (Davies *et al.*, 1995; McMorris, 2004; Schmidt, 1991; Schmidt and Wrisberg, 2000). Reaction time can be sub-divided into pre-motor time and motor time. Pre-motor time is the time from the presentation of the stimulus until muscle activation at the neuromuscular junction, and motor time is the time from muscle activation at the neuromuscular junction to the beginning of the movement (Ketcham and Stelmach, 2004).

A range of different stimuli exists in the sports environment, and sometimes all the performer has to respond to is a single stimulus, such as the starting gun in a sprint race. This is known as simple reaction time (SRT), where there is only one stimulus and the same response is required every time. However, there are times when a response to more than one stimulus is required, such as the kick boxer having to respond to either a kick or a punch, and having to make an effective block with either their arm or leg. This is known as choice reaction time (CRT), when there is more than one stimulus present to which a correct response has to be made.

One of the most important laws in human performance was discovered by Hick and Hyman in 1952 and 1953 respectively, who found there was a linear relationship between CRT and the number of stimulus response alternatives. The relationship implies that CRT increases at a constant rate of around 150 milliseconds (McMorris, 2004) every time the number of stimulus response alternatives is doubled (Schmidt, 1991; Schmidt and Wrisberg, 2000).

However, there are issues when two stimuli are presented very close together, e.g. the rugby player dropping their shoulder to fake a move one way only to go the other (selling a dummy). When two stimuli are presented close together the reaction time to the second stimulus is slower than the normal reaction time (Welford, 1968) and this is called the psychological refractory period (PRP). This is thought to occur because the individual cannot process the information from the second stimulus until the first stimulus has been dealt with (McMorris, 2004).

FEEDBACK

Feedback can be defined as the return of information about the result of skill execution. Schmidt (1991) suggests there are two main sources of feedback: intrinsic feedback (sometimes called inherent feedback) and extrinsic feedback (sometimes called augmented feedback).

Intrinsic feedback comes from sensory information outside of the body (exteroception) or from within the body (proprioception) (Schmidt and Wrisberg, 2000). For example, the high jumper would feel the rush of air around their body as they are making the run up to the bar (exteroception), and feel the plant of the take-off foot and flexion of muscles on take-off (proprioception).

Extrinsic feedback consists of information that is provided by an external source (Foxon, 2001; Schmidt and Wrisberg, 2000). For example, external sources include the coach providing instructional feedback, showing a DVD of a gymnastics routine or a passage of play in a rugby match, or the performer using a golf score card or recording 3000 m steeplechase lap times.

Both sources can provide the following types of information: knowledge of results (KR), which is information regarding the outcome of an action, and knowledge of performance (KP), which is information about the movement itself (Foxon, 2001).

There are two other considerations in the provision of feedback: bandwidth and the fading technique. Bandwidth feedback involves the coach only giving feedback when the individual movements fall outside some acceptable level of correctness (Schmidt and Wrisberg, 2000). The easiest way to explain this is to use the example of a golfer on the putting green. If the coach has set a target of the putt to be within 30 cm (one foot) of the hole, he would only give feedback if the ball lands outside of the target range. The golfer would then know that he or she would have to exert slightly more force on the putt to ensure that the ball stops within the intended target range.

The fading technique is generally just reducing the frequency of feedback as the performer becomes more skilled in executing the task (McMorris, 2004). Winstein and Schmidt (1990) found that faded feedback achieved more improved retention on motor skill learning. As the coach becomes more confident and experienced, the feedback that they provide to the performer will be less frequent but the quality will be a lot higher.

A further issue regarding the provision of feedback is that of reinforcement, of which there are two types: positive reinforcement, which is the coach providing specific feedback on correct performance execution (Schmidt, 1991) and negative reinforcement, which is not dissimilar to positive reinforcement and is not punishment (Schmidt and Wrisberg, 2000). An example of the latter might be the coach for a period of time providing negative comments on continuous poor skill execution. After being subjected to these negative comments, the performer then executes the skill correctly. Another example might be the coach keeping quiet and not offering any reinforcement of correct skill execution, thereby covertly reinforcing correct skill execution.

Some coaches see punishment as being a reinforcing technique – nothing could be further from the truth, because doing shuttle runs serves no purpose if the performers do not execute what is being asked of them effectively. All the coach is doing is attaching a negative response to poorly executed technique. Feedback should be constructive, and constructive feedback has been shown to be effective whether it is positive or negative (McMorris, 2004). It is recommended that rather than use negative comments like "That is poor", "That is wrong" the coach should re-frame their language so that it is more positive, e.g. "Try moving your body this way" or "How could you execute the skill more effectively?" It is a question of communicating effectively, allowing the performer to think about the skill and to take more ownership of their learning.

TYPES OF PRACTICE

Chapter 6 focused on how to structure practice from a practical perspective. This next section will highlight issues concerning the variability of practice from a skill acquisition perspective. Practice is essential if learning is to take place (McMorris and Hale, 2006) and the type of practice schedule that the coach decides to use can impact upon learning. The first type of practice to be considered is massed practice, which is where the intervals between trials of the task are shorter than the time taken to complete one trial (Schmidt, 1991). Massed practice should be used under the following conditions:

- The skill to be learned can be easily performed and mastered quickly.
- Motivation to continue to learn the skill is high.
- The purpose is to simulate fatigued conditions experienced in a game.
- Little time is available to learn the skills needed to perform in the next game.
- The performers are in a later stage of learning, and physical conditioning is high.

(Adapted from Magill, 1993; McMorris, 2004; McMorris and Hale, 2006; Schmidt, 1991; Schmidt and Lee, 1999; Schmidt and Wrisberg, 2000)

However, with this type of practice boredom and fatigue can set in (McMorris, 2004), therefore the coach has to consider the conditions in which he or she wants to set up the practice.

Spaced or distributed practice is where the interval between trials is greater than the time it takes for one trial to be completed, and is interspersed with rest periods and breaks (Schmidt, 1991). Spaced or distributed practice can sometimes lead to better performance, however, following a rest, tests show there is no difference in retention (McMorris, 2004). Spaced or distributed practice is preferred under the following conditions:

- learning a new complex skill
- learning a skill demanding high mental and physical effort
- fatigue causing athletes to learn incorrect motor patterns
- short attention span
- low motivation to learn the skill
- athletes insufficiently conditioned for repetitive performance
- hot and humid conditions.

(Adapted from Magill, 1993; McMorris, 2004; McMorris and Hale, 2006; Schmidt, 1991; Schmidt and Lee, 1999; Schmidt and Wrisberg, 2000)

Two other types of practice warrant explanation: blocked and random practice. Blocked practice is where the learner practices one skill continually before moving onto the next skill; random practice is where the performer practices two or more skills, and has random trials on each skill (Schmidt, 1991). Shea and Morgan (1979) and Goode and Magill (1986) have shown that blocked practice leads to more effective practice performance, but random practice, even though less effective during practice, is better for learning and retention. Green et al. (1995) have also found that random practice is superior to blocked practice, and more recently Reid *et al.* (2006, p. 1) added weight to this contention by suggesting "that players stand to benefit from the earlier introduction of variable and random practices".

The message for the coach is to ensure that practices are varied, and that they do not "drill for drilling's sake" (blocked practice), because although there may be learning taking place during the session, the ability for the performers to retain the skill may be limited. The coach can still focus on a skill theme in order to "groove" the skill, but associated practices should be varied.

The amount of practice (deliberate practice) that a performer carries out is thought to be associated with expert performance. Ericsson *et al.* (1993) suggest that it takes 10,000 hours to become an expert performer, and further studies in figure skating (Starkes *et al.*, 1996), wrestling (Hodges and Starkes, 1996; Starkes *et al.*, 1996), soccer, field hockey (Helson *et al.*, 1998) and martial arts (Hodges and Deakin, 1998 cited in Starkes and Ericsson, 2003) have gone some way to supporting this contention.

However, there are factors that may influence whether these performers reach expert performance, such as finances, the coach, parental support, learner motivation, access to facilities, etc. Moreover, there is no accounting for natural talent and it could be argued that some performers reach expert performance well before the suggested 10,000 hours or 10 years of deliberate practice, and equally there are others who can practise all they like for many years and still not achieve expert status.

A further consideration regarding practice is the transfer of training, which can be divided into two types. Positive transfer of training is where the practice of one task has a facilitative effect on the learning of another; negative transfer is where practice of one task has an inhibiting effect on another (McMorris, 2004; McMorris and Hale, 2006). For example, a positive transfer of training would be the chest pass in basketball and netball, as each requires execution of the same movement patterns. An example of negative transfer of training might be the skills of hitting a hockey ball and swinging a baseball bat, in which the movement patterns are completely different.

SUMMARY

Having a good understanding of how the performer acquires skills is essential for the coach. Skill is classified along four continua, which include open to closed, fine to gross, externally paced to self-paced, and continuous through to serial and discrete. Athletes possess a range of abilities and it is debated whether these abilities are either specific or unique or exist in clusters of abilities.

Different perspectives exist to explain the way in which performers learn, and one of the most enduring notions is Fitts and Posner's (1967) stages of learning, which are the cognitive, associative and autonomous stages. It is also suggested that we learn at both implicit (subconscious) and explicit (learning by instruction) levels. Eysenck and Keane (2005) suggest that memory can be represented as a multi-store system and that three systems exist, the SS, the STM and the LTM. Generally, it is thought that the SS and the STM can only hold information for a very short period of time, and if it is not reinforced then it will not be committed to LTM. Selective attention is the ability to pick out relevant cues in the environment, and it is crucial that the sports person recognizes the correct patterns exhibited by an opponent so that they can execute a correct response. Decision making is in part associated with the ability to scan the visual field effectively (Knudson and Kluka,

1997) to learn what is relevant or irrelevant (selective attention) and in part associated with our perceptual abilities, i.e. the performer tries to make sense of the information that is presented to them. Being able to anticipate quickly and effectively is an huge advantage in sports performance, and allows the performer to make a decision and respond to it quickly. Anticipation can be defined as the ability to have an expectation of, or to predict upcoming events in the visual field.

Reaction time is the speed at which we make decisions, and two types of reaction time are said to exist: the Simple Reaction Time (SRT) and Choice Reaction Time (CRT). SRT is when there is only one stimulus and the same response is required each time, and CRT is when there is more than one stimulus present.

It is suggested that without practice we cannot and will not learn, and feedback helps us learn faster and more accurately (McMorris, 2004). There are two main sources of feedback: intrinsic feedback (sometimes called inherent feedback) and extrinsic feedback (sometimes called augmented feedback). Intrinsic feedback comes from sensory information outside of the body (exteroception) or from within the body (proprioception). Structuring practice is a fundamental part of the coaching process and it is essential if learning is to take place. Practices must be varied, and the type of practice schedule that the coach decides to use can have an impact upon learning.

SEMINAR OR DISCUSSION QUESTIONS

1. Choose a range of sports and sports skills and identify how they would be classified on the skill classification continua.
2. Identify how you would structure practice in a sport of your choice for:

- a novice group
- an expert group
- a group which has a big game or performance at the weekend, and you only have two days to instruct a new skill or tactic.

KEY TERMS AND DEFINITIONS

- Ability – basic innate actions that underlie skilled performance.
- Anticipation – ability to have an expectation of or to predict upcoming events in the visual field.
- Decision making – knowing what to do, when to do it and how to do it.
- Feedback – return of information about the result of skill execution.
- Learning – a relatively permanent change in performance.
- Long-term memory – holds information for long periods of time.
- Reaction time – the speed at which we make decisions.
- Selective attention – ability to pick out relevant cues in the environment.
- Sensory store – holds information for around 250 milliseconds.
- Short-term memory – holds information for around 30 seconds.

- Skill – the ability to bring about pre-determined results with maximum certainty, often with the minimum outlay of time, energy or both.
- Variability of practice – use of different practice schedules to facilitate the learning process.

WEB LINKS

Skill acquisition – www.brianmac.co.uk

FURTHER READING

Ericsson, K. A., Krampe, R. T., and Tesch-Romer, C. (1993). The role of deliberate practice in the acquisition of expert performance. *Psychological Review*. 100, 363–406.

Hodges, N. J. and Starkes, J. L. (1996). Wrestling with the nature of expertise: A sport specific test of Ericsson, Krampe and Tesch-Romer's (1993) Theory of 'deliberate practice'. *International Journal of Sport Psychology*, 27, 400–24.

Helson, W. F., Starkes, J. L., and Hodges, N. J. (1998). Team sports and the theory of deliberate practice. *Journal of Sport and Exercise Psychology*, 20. 12–34.

Honeybourne, J. (2006). *Acquiring Skill in Sport: An Introduction*. Routledge, London.

Magill, R. A. (1993). *Motor Learning: Concepts and Applications*. McGraw-Hill, New York

McMorris, T. (2004). *Acquisition and Performance of Sports Skills*. Wiley & Sons, Chichester.

McMorris, T. and Hale, T. (2006). *Coaching Science; Theory into Practice*. Wiley & Sons, Chichester.

Schmidt, R. A. (1991). *Motor Learning and Performance: From Principles to Practice*. Human Kinetics, Champaign, IL.

Schmidt, R. A. and Wrisberg, C. A. (2000). *Motor Learning and Performance: A Problem Based Learning Approach*. Human Kinetics, Champaign, IL.

Starkes, J. L., Deakin, J., Allard, F., Hodges, N. J. and Hayes, A. (1996). Deliberate practice in sports: What is it anyway? In K. A. Ericsson (ed.) *The road to excellence: The acquisition of expert performance in the arts and sciences, sports, and games*. Erlbaum, Mahwah, NJ, 81–106.

Starkes, J. L. and Ericsson, K. A. (2003). *Expert Performance in Sports: Advances in Research on Sport Expertise*. Human Kinetics, Champaign, IL.

Chapter 15

Biomechanics, performance analysis and the coach

CHAPTER OBJECTIVES

■ Outline basic principles of biomechanics.
■ Identify and describe types of technology that can aid the coach.
■ Outline and explain the use of notational analysis.

BASIC BIOMECHANICS

Biomechanics is the scientific discipline concerned with the forces acting on the athlete and the effects produced by these forces (Bartlett, 1997, 1999). At high level sport, precise technique execution is critical, and the best performance improvement and adjustment comes from careful attention to detail (Hall, 2007; Hay, 1993). It is therefore crucial that the coach has a good understanding of biomechanics.

Biomechanics can be sub-divided into kinematics, kinetics, anthropometrics and kinesiology. Kinematics is the study of the description of motion, including considerations of space and time; kinetics is the study of the action of forces; anthropometrics is related to the dimensions and weights of body segments (Hall, 2007); and kinesiology is the study of human movement, which can also be described as functional anatomy (covered in Chapter 10). In order to simplify the concept of biomechanics, this chapter will be stay very much at a fundamental level, and only the basic concepts will be highlighted. Moreover, the chapter will not include any line drawings to describe typical concepts in human movement. For more in-depth coverage and line drawings of fundamental movement principles of biomechanics, see the suggested further reading at the end of this chapter which is for both the coach and student.

Motion

Linear motion is where an object or group of objects uniformly moves in the same direction, form and speed, and is also known as translatory motion (Hall, 2007). For example, the ski jumper experiences translation of motion in flight after lifting off from the jump ramp. They glide in the same direction, form and speed through the air prior to landing. Linear motion can either be straight (rectilinear), e.g. the snow boarder going down a slope in a straight line, or curved (curvilinear), e.g. the snow boarder carrying out a specific routine in a half-pipe.

Angular motion or rotation occurs when all parts of the body move through the same angle but do not undergo the same linear displacement (Hamill and Knutzen, 1995). An example is the gymnast on the asymmetric bars performing a full rotation, or the swimmer performing a tumble turn in a swimming race.

However, human movement usually consists of general motion rather than pure linear or angular motion (Bartlett, 1995; Hall, 2007; Hay, 1993). For example, the runner, cyclist or swimmer will move in a straight line, with all the different body parts rotating at the joints.

Linear and angular kinematics

Kinematics is concerned with the form of motion with respect to time, and is inclusive of distance, displacement, speed, velocity and acceleration (Hall, 2007; Hay, 1995). It can be sub-divided into linear (straight line) and angular (rotation of body parts) kinematics. Distance is the length of the path the body follows and displacement (linear and angular) is the length of the path "as the crow flies". For example, the distance of a running road race may be 10 km, but in a straight line the displacement may only be 8km, which is the distance the runner has actually displaced between the start and finish points.

The rate at which a body moves from one location to another is known as speed. Speed is not velocity; speed is found by dividing the distance covered by the time taken, and velocity (linear and angular) is found by dividing the displacement by the time taken (Bartlett, 1999). Acceleration (linear and angular) is the rate of change in velocity (Hay, 1995).

Linear and angular kinetics

Kinetics is concerned with the causes of motion and is sub-divided into either linear or angular kinetics. The concept of force must be considered when examining the effects of kinetic linear motion (Hamill and Knutzen, 1995). A force can be thought of as the pushing and pulling action that one object exerts on another (Bartlett, 1995).

Force can be further sub-divided into weight, reaction force, buoyancy, impact force, linear, planar and spatial forces, concurrent force, parallel force and general force. Force is not always applied in a linear, uniform fashion; there are many times when force is applied from a rotational (angular) perspective. When a force causes rotation, the rotation occurs at a pivot point, and the line of action of the force must act at a distance from the pivot point (Bartlett, 1999). The best example that can be provided is of the gymnast rotating on the asymmetric bars or rings. They perform a rotation by holding on to the bar or rings and rotating the body extended in a straight line, and it is this rotation that causes force to be applied in the body. The product of that force and the perpendicular distance to its line of action is referred to as a torque or moment of force (Bartlett, 1997).

Newton's laws are also applied in the context of sports biomechanics:

- The law of inertia states that an object will continue in a state of rest or of uniform motion in a straight line unless acted upon by external forces that are not in equilibrium.
- The law of acceleration states that a force applied to a body causes an acceleration of that body of a magnitude proportional to the force, in the direction of the force and inversely proportional to the body's mass.
- The law of reaction states for every action there is an equal and opposite reaction.
(Bartlett, 1995; Hall, 2007; Hamill and Knutzen, 1995; Hay, 1993)

When an object is at rest it is reluctant to do anything and a moving object is also reluctant to change what it is doing. This reluctance to change is called inertia (Hay, 1993). Inertia is directly measured or expressed by the mass of the object, and momentum is the quantity of motion possessed by a body measured by the product of its mass and velocity of its mass centre (Bartlett, 1995).

Projectile trajectory

Three factors influence the trajectory (flight path) of a projectile: the angle of projection, the projection speed and the relative height of projection (Hamill and Knutzen, 1995). Understanding these concepts is useful within the context of sport for understanding how best to project balls and other implements (javelin, discus, shot put) and for predicting how to best catch or strike balls (Hall, 2007).

The angle of projection is defined as the angle between the projectile's velocity vector and the horizontal at the instant of release or take-off, hence the terms "release angle" or "take-off angle" are often used (Bartlett, 1995). Projection speed determines the length or size of a projectile's trajectory (Hall, 2007) and the projection height is the difference in height between the vertical take-off position and the vertical landing position (Hall, 2007; Hamill and Knutzen, 1995).

Friction

Friction is a force that acts at the surfaces of an object in the opposite direction to the direction of motion or imminent motion (Hall, 2007). Friction can be sub-divided into maximum static friction, which is the maximum amount of friction that can be generated between two static surfaces, and kinetic friction, which is friction generated between two surfaces in contact during motion, such as a field hockey ball rolling along AstroTurf.

Centre of gravity

The coach should have a good understanding of centre of gravity (CoG) principles because changes in CoG can determine balance and influence the performer's ability to execute some skills. When standing upright, our CoG is an imaginary line through the centre of our body, and as we move our bodies in time and space our CoG changes. For example, the pole vaulter's CoG will change numerous times as they are going through the approach phase, the planting of the pole, kicking up and through with the legs, pushing down on the pole to get the extra lift to get the body over the bar and the eventual dropping down to the safety mat.

Anthropometrics

Anthropometrics is the study of the human body in terms of measuring different body parts (arms and legs) and properties (body mass) to assist in understanding the variations that exist in different body types (Bartlett, 1995). For example, the mass of each body segment and the segment's centre of mass position can be used in calculating the position of the whole body centre of mass (Bartlett, 1995). Many advanced techniques exist for taking measures of body segments but a simple one is called the immersion method, whereby the individual puts his or her limb into a large container of water. The water that has overflowed and been displaced is collected and then weighed to provide the volume of the segment.

TECHNOLOGY, PERFORMANCE ANALYSIS AND THE COACH

A major problem facing the coach is the issue of objectivity when coaching skills and analysing performance. It is impossible for the coach to be able to recall all events that take place in training and competition. Therefore accurate measures and measuring systems are necessary for effective feedback and improvement of performance (Hughes, 2004). Technology can aid performance analysis by eliminating subjective assessments of performance. Franks and Miller (1986) found that soccer coaches were less than 45 per cent correct in post-game assessments of what occurred during the first 45 minutes of a soccer game, which highlights the issue of accurate objective assessment.

The science of performance analysis has made extraordinary advances in recent years, and different forms of technology are now being used to support the analysis process. Twenty years ago, heart rate monitors were a new concept in providing data on sports performance, but are now a standard item in the coach's toolkit (Drawer, 2006). Bulky video cameras were widely used a decade or so ago, but the majority were unwieldy to use and the playback facility on most was not that refined. Now handheld digital cameras are being used by many coaches as a performance analysis tool.

Sport has benefited from technology that has been around for some time, and some of the technical advances that have been made by the military and the medical and motor car industries have been adapted by sports scientists and coaches for sport performance analysis (Drawer, 2006). These adaptations include physiological and biomechanical measurement technology and advances in material construction, which is pushing the boundaries in equipment design. For example, scientists are adding technological improvements to running shoes, making them springier by providing greater "energy return". Increasingly flexible

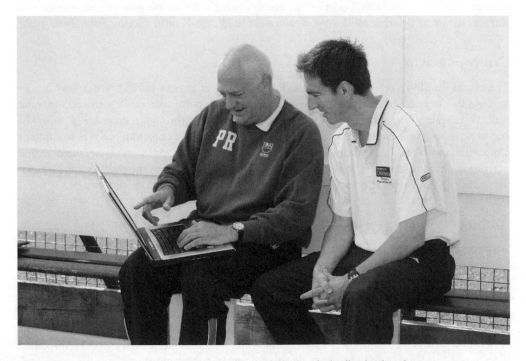

Photo 15.1 A coach using a laptop as a coaching aid to provide feedback of performance.

carbon-fibre vaulting poles have sent records tumbling, and in archery arrows of composite materials go farther, faster and straighter (Connor, 2000).

As well as technological advances in equipment design, there are a range of technological tools available to the coach for performance analysis purposes and these include:

- Digitization – a process by which reflective markers are placed on selected joints and limbs of a performer. The performer is then filmed executing a particular skill. The film is then taken back to the laboratory, where the image of the performer is replaced by a line drawing, which corresponds with the reflective markers to enable the performance analyst to observe a range of movements and joint angles.
- Digital cameras – useful in capturing real-time performance and playback.
- DVD players – more versatile than video players, because the coach is able to select an action frame by frame without the blurring that was evident when using video. Also, picture quality is of a higher definition when using DVDs.
- Digital versatile cameras – cameras are on the market that can burn a disc within the camera, so the coach is able to take the disc away instantaneously and play it back on a DVD player or laptop computer.
- Helmet cameras – small versatile cameras that can transmit a signal back to a laptop and are used in canoeing, rock climbing, etc.
- Laptop computers – these are becoming more portable and have longer battery lives and increased hard drive memory capability.
- A range of PC software performer analysis packages exist such as Sportscode, Prozone, Kandle, Qunitex and Gamebreaker, which can analyse an individual performer's actions, position or distance covered. However, many of these packages are being increasingly used in the team environment, where, for example, distance covered, pattern of movement, types of run, percentage of passes made and tackles won are being analysed. This information is useful to the coach because they can also analyse the opposition's strengths and weaknesses, so the coach can then structure training accordingly.

Other technological advances in performance analysis include:

- Core temperature measurement – a small pill is swallowed (temperature sensor) and once it is in the gut, temperature data is wirelessly transmitted to the logging unit attached to the body. Skin temperature patches are now also being used.
- Multiple heart rate transmission – previously the coach or sports scientist was only able to measure individual heart rates. Equipment now exists that provides simultaneous wireless heart rate transmission for up to 32 people over a stated range of 200 m.
- Distance, position, time, speed, altitude and heart rate – global positioning satellite (GPS) technology is being used to track and analyse the performer's movement.
- Real-time visual feedback – heads-up display units (HUD) provide the coach and performer with the ability to transmit video or numerical data in real time on the inside of goggles through wireless transmission.
- Audio coach feedback – in some sports, where feedback is hindered by noise such as Formula One car racing, technology has enabled noise cancelling transmission to ensure that the message has not been lost. Noise cancelling helmets provide the opportunity for better quality feedback.

(Drawer, 2006)

NOTATIONAL ANALYSIS

Notational analysis is used by coaches and sport scientists to gather objective data on the performance of athletes. Notational analysis methods are becoming increasingly refined, which reflects the demands of coaches and scientists, as well as the desire to statistically analyse performance in order to gain a competitive edge (Hughes and Franks, 2004). Tactics, technique, individual athlete movement and work rate can all be analysed, enabling coaches and athletes to learn more about performance, and at the same time this provides an extrinsic source of feedback for the performer. Many of the software packages outlined in the previous section are also used as notational analysis systems in order to provide accurate feedback to the performer.

Although a range of technology is available to the coach, there is sometimes no substitute for the use of paper and pencil when analysing performance, which is a simple and effective method to use. The coach should find a method that suits them and is fit for the purpose, in terms of identifying what kind of information they want to gain from conducting the analysis. Tally charts are a simple method of analysis available to the coach, e.g. the team sports coach could count the number of successful passes made in a passage of play or a whole game. If the percentage of successful passes were low, then possibly there could be an issue of retention of possession, which could be addressed in the next training session. An example of a notational analysis form for field hockey is given in Appendix 12.

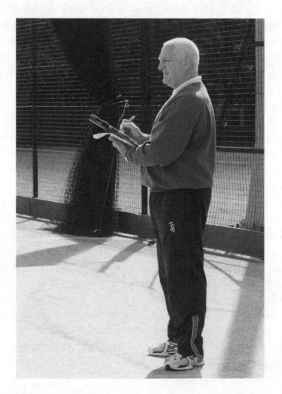

Photo 15.2 A coach using notational analysis.

SUMMARY

It is essential that the coach has a fundamental understanding of the processes and principles that underpin human movement. Biomechanics is the scientific discipline concerned with the forces acting on the athlete and the effects produced by these forces (Bartlett, 1997, 1999), and can be sub-divided into kinematics, kinetics, anthropometrics and kinesiology. Sport is not motionless and it is therefore essential that the coach have a good understanding of how and why the performer moves.

Motion can be described as linear (moving in a straight line) and angular (rotational), and two sub-disciplines exist in biomechanics that serve to explain motion. Kinematics is concerned with the description of motion and kinetics is concerned with the causes of motion, both of which have a linear and angular component. Understanding how best to project balls and other implements (javelin, discus, shot put) and predicting how to best catch or strike projected balls and gauge their trajectory are essential. For example, the javelin coach will coach his or her performer to release the javelin at the optimum moment, and help the performer to understand that the angle of the body and javelin at release is a crucial factor in determining distance thrown.

Three factors influence the trajectory (flight path) of a projectile: the angle of projection, the projection speed and the relative height of projection (Hamill and Knutzen, 1995). The coaching of skills depends significantly upon analysis to effect an improvement in performance, and informed and accurate measures are necessary for effective feedback and improvement of performance (Hughes, 2004). Technological advances have provided the coach with a range of tools to support the performance analysis process. However, although this technology is readily available to the coach, there is sometimes no substitute for pencil and paper notational analysis techniques, which can provide meaningful data and information.

SEMINAR OR DISCUSSION QUESTIONS

1. Identify a technological tool that is available to the coach and describe how it could be useful analysing performance in a sport of your choice.
2. Construct a pencil and paper notational analysis sheet which can provide meaningful data and information in a sport of your choice.

KEY TERMS AND DEFINITIONS

- Angular – involving rotation around a central line or point.
- Anthropometric – related to the dimensions and weights of body segments.
- Centre of gravity – point around which a body's weight is equally balanced.
- Digitization – a performance analysis process.
- Force – push or pull; the product of mass and acceleration.
- Friction – force acting on the area of contact between two surfaces in the opposite direction to that of motion or impending motion.
- General motion – motion inclusive of translation and rotation simultaneously.

- Inertia – tendency of a body to resist change in its state of motion.
- Kinematics – form, pattern or sequencing of movement with respect to time.
- Kinesiology – study of human movement.
- Kinetics – study of the action of forces.
- Linear – along a line, straight or curved, with all parts of the body moving in the same direction at the same speed.
- Mass – quantity of matter contained in an object.
- Notational analysis – process used to gather objective data on the performance of athletes.
- Projection speed – the magnitude of projection velocity.
- Rectilinear – along a straight line.
- Torque – the rotary effect of force about an axis of rotation.
- Trajectory – flight path of a projectile.

WEB LINKS

General biomechanics – www.brianmac.co.uk
Sport technology – www.minimitter.com
– www.hosand.com
– www.gpsports.com
– www.headzone.com.au
– www.roboprobe.com

FURTHER READING

Bartlett, R. (1997). *Introduction to Sports Biomechanics*. Routledge, London.
Bartlett, R. (1999). *Sports Biomechanics*. Routledge, London.
Grimshaw, P., Lees, A., Fowler, N. and Burden, A. (2006). *Instant Notes in Sport and Exercise Biomechanics*. Routledge, London.
Hall, S. B. (2007). *Basic Biomechanics*. McGraw-Hill, London.
Hamill, J. and Knutzen, K. M. (1995). *Biomechanical Basis of Human Movement*. Williams and Wilkins, London.
Hay, J. G (1993). *The Biomechanics of Sports Techniques* (4th edn). Prentice-Hall, Englewood Cliffs, NJ.
Hughes, M. (2004). Performance analysis – a 2004 perspective. *International Journal of Performance Analysis in Sport*, 4, 1, 96–103.
Hughes, M. and Franks, I. (2004). *Notational Analysis of Sport: Systems for Better Coaching and Performance in Sport*. Routledge, England.
Hong, Y. and Bartlett, R. (2008). *Routledge Handbook of Biomechanics and Human Movement Science*. Routledge, London.
SportsCoachUK (2006). On the pulse: Cutting edge technology for coaches. *Coaching Edge*, 4, 10–33.

Part 6

Further considerations for the coach

INTRODUCTION

This, the final part of this book will concentrate on further considerations for the coach. The content of this part should not be seen as an exhaustive list of things that the coach should further consider in their day-to-day coaching practice, but as a demonstration for the coach that there are many other aspects associated with the practice of coaching.

Chapter 16 explores and highlights the importance of coach education and the coach educator, and the role that GBoS have in developing coach education programmes. A case study is provided of a practising coach educator who holds a senior position at SportsCoachUK. Coaches also need to be developed and mentored through their coaching qualifications, therefore Chapter 16 also outlines the importance of the mentoring process.

Chapter 17 explores the issues of working with special populations. The role of the coach coaching children and their child protection responsibilities are examined in depth. The Long Term Athlete Development Programme has been taken up by a number of sports in the UK, and this concept is outlined. The different stages of development that have been proposed by Istvan Balyi and colleagues are identified and described. Coaching the disabled performer is also outlined in Chapter 17, highlighting the inclusivity aspect of accessibility to high quality coaching and how the coach can adapt coaching practice.

Chapter 18 examines the issues of lifestyle management and the role of the coach. Many athletes make sacrifices to excel in their chosen sport, but this is sometimes to the detriment of family, education, employment and financial opportunities and therefore the importance of a balanced lifestyle is addressed. Use of performance enhancing drugs and supplementation and the role of the coach are also covered in Chapter 18.

The final chapter, Chapter 19, explains the concepts of talent identification and talent transfer. The coach will on a regular basis have to select athletes to be part of a squad or a team and some coaches may find themselves in a position that requires them to talent-spot promising athletes. Therefore having an understanding of the processes involved is useful. Furthermore, the concept of talent transfer is becoming more prominent, with athletes transferring their talent from one sport to another, and this concept is also explained in Chapter 19. At the end of each chapter suggested seminar or discussion questions and key terms and definitions are provided in order to support student learning. Web links and further reading are also provided in order for the student to carry out further research if required.

Chapter 16

Coach education and mentoring

CHAPTER OBJECTIVES

- Highlight the coach education process.
- Provide a case study of the development of a coach educator.
- Explain coach mentoring.

COACH EDUCATION

Coach education and development is central to the professionalization of sports coaching (Lyle, 2007). Moreover, coach education and development is essential in order for a critical mass of coaches to be harnessed in the UK to support athletes at whatever level they perform. In order to achieve this critical mass, an accessible, quality assured and clear coach development pathway system needs to exist.

One of the aims of the UK Coaching Framework is to provide systems that support the coaching process at all levels (SportsCoachUK, 2008l), and coach education is a critical component of a coaching support system. SportsCoachUK and GBoS have developed and implemented a range of initiatives, services, courses and resources that support coach education, and GBoS now have clearly defined coach development and coach educator development pathways in place in sports such as cricket, field hockey and swimming.

An individual starting out in their coaching career more often than not starts at the beginner level, and will need to attend a GBoS Level 1 Coach Award. Scarth *et al.* (2008) suggest that obtaining a qualification results in a learner reaching a "Training Performance Standard, which is the minimum level required to be awarded the qualification, but coach education needs to move learners to Operational Performance Standard, which is a higher level of coaching proficiency: qualifications are a step on the journey of developing expertise; a qualification is not the journey" (Scarth *et al.* 2008).

The coach must not think that their education stops when they receive their Coach Award qualification; they should seek out other learning experiences to further expand and challenge their knowledge and beliefs. Coaching is an ongoing, fluid, ever changing and reflective learning process. The coach should engage in "horizontal learning" and attend GBoS workshops or short courses, coaching conferences and keep up to date with first aid, insurance, child protection certification and any other courses or events that are relevant to their development. Also, the coach should access a range of learning resources, observe other coaches to gain experience of different ways that coaches deliver and coach as much as they can to gain practice experience.

A system has been developed in the UK whereby young bright and forward thinking coaches can be identified and given the opportunity to be fast tracked to work with the nation's top athletes. UK Sport is delivering a programme called "Elite Coach" (UK Sport, 2008a), which is designed to fast track the development of coaches who have the potential to provide the best possible coaching for Great Britain's top athletes, thus providing the best chance of success in London 2012. Individual programmes are developed for each coach and their specific needs, which allow them to develop both their technical and tactical skills by working with and observing the best in action (UK Sport, 2008a).

The coach educator plays a pivotal role in developing coaches and many give up their time at weekends to tutor coaching courses. The coach educator is generally a senior experienced coach, and certain criteria have to be met and certain courses attended before one can tutor and assess on Coach Award courses. A large part of the tutor training programme is usually organized and delivered by the GBoS, but certain elements are also delivered by SportsCoachUK coach educator tutor training staff. Some GBoS have a career path in place for coach educators, which is similar to that of the candidate coach progressing through the Coach Award scheme.

An example of good practice is given by England Hockey, where a robust and quality assured coach education programme exists that has set criteria that have to be met by the coach educator before they can tutor and assess on coaching courses. For example, the Level 1 Coach Award head tutor has to attend a Safeguarding and Protection course, have a current first aid certificate, attend an annual generic tutor assessor training event and Certificate in Tutoring in Sport workshops, tutor a minimum of one course per year, and attend a minimum of two CPD events and one regional workshop covering technique and/or tactics each year (Baker, 2007).

To tutor on a Level 1 Coach Award the tutor has to be at least a Level 2 coach, and to tutor a Level 2 Coach Award the tutor has to be at least a Level 3 coach (Baker, 2006), and so forth up to the Level 4 Coach Award. On top of this there is an ongoing trainee coach education system in place in order to recruit potential coach educators. The systems and processes that England Hockey has put in place are rigorous, but the quality of coach education is thereby raised and robust; formal and distinct pathways exist for the coach and coach educator.

Case study 17.1 – The coach educator

Mark is an England Hockey Level 3 coach and a senior coach educator who started coaching in 1982. He has been a coach educator for ten years and is currently a trainee National Trainer for SportsCoachUK, as well as being employed by SportsCoachUK as their South East England Regional Manager. Mark's first coaching role was for a Royal Air Force Ladies Station side in 1982. He coached as a volunteer until around 1996, at which time he decided to take his role as a coach more seriously, progressing to club coaching at gradually higher levels.

Although he gained his Level 1 Coach Award in 1992 and had progressed to Level 3 by 1996, between 1982 and 1998 he received little encouragement to develop himself as a coach. Around 1996 Mark expressed a desire to become a coach educator and qualified as a coach educator for Levels 1 and 2 in 1998. He has progressed to become a senior coach tutor, which has also been facilitated by his working for SportsCoachUK since 2004. Mark's philosophy as a coach educator is to give each individual as much as he can, depending on the stage of their development. When tutoring Mark is conscious that he must cater for all individuals' needs, which at times can be problematic because some information that he provides is additional to the curriculum. However, he feels that this additional information is important and relevant to the needs of the candidate, depending on the situation that they find themselves in. Mark is also determined to make coach education relevant to the individual's world, and emphasizes that coaching is about learning and improvement, suggesting that "we are not in the business of running activity sessions where no learning takes place". Mark takes a view that he is responsible for maximizing the potential of all his athletes and his trainee coaches.

Mark thinks that coach education is at a crossroads in the UK, and since the introduction of the UKCC there is a perception that coach education is more expensive. However, his personal view is that quality costs, and for too long we have been looking at coach education as a numbers game, which has to be tempered. We need to look at quality and start to think about lifelong learning, which could develop as a result of the UK Coaching Framework. Mark thinks that there are exciting times ahead and if we can get it right then we can move forward with coaching in the UK.

He believes that mentoring and the provision of informal cross-sport learning opportunities are two of the most important aspects of coach education, together with the long-term development of the coach in developing expertise. Moreover, critical to the success of coach education is the provision of ongoing support after a qualification has been taken. Mark views the mentor as having a massive role to play in the facilitation of learning (whole person learning). The role of the mentor is to facilitate the provision of what the learner needs at that stage of their development. This means that as a mentor you do not have to be an expert in a specific sport, but you do need to be an expert in recognizing stages of development. Any coach can source technical and tactical specialists as and when required. Mark continues to work in coach education and is passionate in driving coaching and the quality of coaching forward in the UK.

THE MENTORING PROCESS

Although attending coach education courses increases the knowledge base of the coach, Abrahams and Collins (1998) and Douge *et al.* (1994) suggest that they rarely improve the overall coaching effectiveness of the coach, which is perhaps where the mentor should take a greater role in the coach's development.

"Mentoring is a powerful tool in the education and development of sports coaches at all levels, and successful coach education programmes change the behaviour and practice of coaches, whether they are novices or international coaches" (Galvin, 2003). Mentoring is also a one-to-one relationship supporting the development of another coach, and should be a two-way symbiotic process and a relationship that both the mentor and mentee contribute to. Mentoring is essentially about helping coaches to learn and take responsibility for their own development (Owen, 2003; Parsons, 2005; Still, 2003).

Mentoring is nothing new in sport, and many coaches have turned to a more experienced coach and asked for advice. However, mentoring provides a more formal process by which the coach can learn their "trade". The mentoring process provides a more structured way to guide a coach through what can be a challenging and daunting learning process. Mentoring is a highly effective way for coaches to learn and apply concepts that they may have learnt on a coaching course, and mentors can facilitate this learning process by adding practical coaching skills and solutions to the theoretical content learnt in the class room (ASC, 2008b).

Many organizations in different countries such as Canada and Germany have identified that the most appropriate method of developing effective coaches is through some form of apprenticeship or mentoring programme, and these programmes are integrated into their coach education process (Nash, 2003). In Canada the Coaching Association of Canada has developed a systematic mentoring process which recognizes three fundamental approaches to mentoring, providing a supervisory role which is both informal and facilitated (CAC, 2005). After the unification of Germany the German coach education system has encouraged and facilitated mentorship opportunities from participant to elite levels (Nash, 2003).

Although much has been written in the UK regarding the effectiveness of mentoring, not all sports have a systematic mentoring process in place. In many sports, "coaches often fulfil the role of mentor, but the role of the coach does not automatically embrace the tasks of a mentor" (Payne et al., 2002, p. 30). SportsCoachUK has commissioned research to critically review the sports coach and wider mentoring literature and evidence, and to undertake new primary work to develop a training package for sports coach mentors (SportsCoachUK, 2008m). SportsCoachUK hopes the results from this research will identify the key components in the mentoring process, and inform the development of a systematic mentoring mechanism, which will further enhance the quality of coaching and coach education in the UK.

There are benefits for the coach, mentor and organization when a mentoring system is in place, which the Australian Sports Commission suggests are as follows:

For the coach

- can increase confidence, motivation and self-fulfilment
- provides objective and constructive feedback on their performance
- helps coaches translate theoretical coaching principles into practice

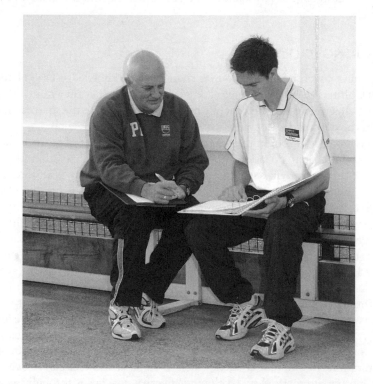

Photo 16.1 A mentor discussing a coaches progress.

- provides opportunities to network, share good practice and further enhance career prospects
- promotes lifelong learning through relationships with other coaches and support networks
- minimizes the difficulties of attending training courses while developing a range of other skill sets (questioning, inviting and providing feedback, etc.) that are associated with coaching practice.

For the mentor

- provides renewed enthusiasm and commitment to the mentor's own coaching practice
- creates opportunities for mentors to share good practice
- it recognizes the expertise, skills and qualities that mentors develop
- provides new opportunities for mentors to learn a range of different skill sets.

For the organization

- eases the cost of lengthy residential courses
- taps into the expertise and skill pool of experienced coaches
- provides a coaching support network
- coaches who have been mentored often become mentors
- encourages coaches to progress to the next Coaching Award.

(ASC, 2008b)

The process of mentoring has the relationship between coach and mentor at its hub (Haskins, 2003), and there are key steps in the process, through which the coach and mentor transit:

- Identifying the needs of the coach.
- Goal setting – setting specific goals to achieve the identified needs.
- Establish an agreement – when and how often to meet, and when to review the relationship.
- Observation – how often and when to observe.
- Analysis and feedback – coach to be given opportunity to analyse and reflect upon performance.
- Action planning – once mentor has observed and analysed, both can explore ways to improve performance.
- Review – the relationship can change and grow and the effectiveness of the relationship as well as coaching performance should be reviewed.

(Adapted from ASC, 2008b; Galvin, 2003; Haskins, 2003)

SUMMARY

It is essential that a highly skilled, qualified and motivated coach education workforce exists to develop coaches in the UK and other countries. The coach should engage in "horizontal learning" and attend GBoS workshops or short courses, coaching conferences, and keep up to date with first aid, insurance, child protection certification and any other courses or events that are relevant to their development. Coach educators are expected to go through a rigorous training and development process themselves in order to be able to deliver coach education courses.

In order to further support coaches, mentoring is useful in bridging the gap between coaching knowledge and coaching effectiveness, and can be a valuable experience to both the mentor and the coach. Mentoring is a one-to-one relationship supporting the development of another coach, and should be a two-way process that both parties should contribute to. Mentoring is essentially about helping coaches to learn and take responsibility for their own development. There are benefits for the coach, mentor and organization when a mentoring system is in place, and there are also key steps in the process that the mentor and the coach should transit such as identifying needs, goal setting, action planning and reviewing the process.

SEMINAR OR DISCUSSION QUESTIONS

1. Identify the coach education pathway in a sport of your choice.
2. Identify the key steps in the mentoring process and apply them in a role play scenario, with one person being the mentor and another being the coach.

KEY TERMS AND DEFINITIONS

- Coach educator – a senior coach who delivers Coach Award courses.
- Mentor – a senior coach who in developing a one-to-one relationship supports the development of another coach.

WEB LINKS

Coach education – www.sportscoachuk.org.
Coach mentoring for women in Canada – www.coach.ca
Coach mentoring in the UK – www.sportscoachuk.org

FURTHER READING

Cushion, C. J. (2006). Mentoring: Harnessing the power of experience. In R. Jones (ed.). *The Sports Coach as Educator: Reconceptualizing Sports Coaching*. Routledge, Oxford.
Galvin, B. (2003). *A Guide to Mentoring Sports Coaches*. Coachwise/SportsCoachUK, Leeds.
Haskin, D. (2003). The mentoring process. *Faster, Higher, Stronger*, 18, 10–11.
Jones, R. l. (2006). *The Sports Coach as an Educator*. Routledge, London.
Owen, M. (2003). Mentoring in context. *Faster, Higher, Stronger*, 18, 7–8.
Still, M. (2003). Why mentoring? *Faster, Higher, Stronger*, 18, 6.

Chapter 17

Coaching special populations

CHAPTER OBJECTIVES

- Outline child protection issues and the role of the coach.
- Highlight the issues coaching children.
- Outline the key elements in the Long Term Athlete Development Programme.
- Highlight the considerations when coaching disabled performers.

CHILD PROTECTION AND THE COACH

"In 2007 over 27,000 children in the UK are on the child protection register, and have suffered with either neglect, physical, sexual or emotional abuse" (NSPCC, 2007). Each week around eight million UK children play sport (Active Surrey, 2008) and unfortunately a small number are at risk from abuse by adults using sport as a vehicle to cause harm. Recent high profile cases in the UK press (a female tennis coach in 2007 and a male gymnastics and trampoline coach in 2008) have unfortunately tarnished sport and coaching. The UN Convention on Children's Human Rights has underpinned work undertaken by sport to address abuse (Boocock, 2007). David (2005 cited in Brackenridge, 2004) sets out five possible sport situations that can threaten the physical and mental integrity of children and has identified the respective articles that are violated:

1. The involvement in intensive training, which is violation of Article 19, protection from child abuse and all forms of violence, and Article 32, protection from economic exploitation.
2. Sexual exploitation, which is violation of Article 19, protection from sexual abuse and violence.
3. Doping, which is violation of Articles 24 and 33, the right to health and protection from drugs.
4. Buying, selling and transfer, which is violation of Article 32, economic exploitation and Article 35, protection from trafficking.
5. Restrictions on education because of involvement in sport, which is violation of Article 28, the right to education.

The Children Act 2004 clearly states that everyone has the responsibility to safeguard the welfare of children and the coach has a duty of care and responsibility when coaching children. Coaches should also be familiar with policies, procedures and legislation that impact upon safeguarding children (Lester, 2003). Sports organizations employing coaches have the same responsibilities, which means:

- A comprehensive child protection policy must exist that is accessible in either paper documentation or electronic means.
- A designated Welfare Officer should be in place having had appropriate training (at the very least they should have attended a child protection workshop, gone through an enhanced Criminal Record Bureau check and had first aid training).
- Policies must exist on recruitment and selection of staff ensuring that appropriate background checks are made, and that staff recruited have the requisite qualifications and experience to match position applied for.
- A written code of behaviour must exist that is available to all coaches, parents and helpers, which may include the Code of Conduct for Sports Coaches, and a Code of Conduct for parents.
- The coach has a training plan (season and session plans) that account for the needs of the children.
- A "whistle blowing" policy must exist.
- A protective culture must exist that accounts for the needs and aspirations of children.
- Policies on bullying, harassment and health and safety should exist, and appropriate risk assessments should be carried out for any potential hazard.
- Robust processes and policies should be in place to deal with concerns and complaints.

(Adapted from Lester, 2003; SSP, 2004)

There are different categories of abuse, such as neglect, physical, sexual and emotional abuse and bullying and harassment. Physical abuse is actual physical violence and can include excessive training loads and regimes or excessive nutritional or weight control; neglect is exposing children to unnecessary risk or harm; sexual abuse is adults or children (male and female) abusing children to satisfy their own sexual desires (Lester, 2003); emotional abuse is constant criticism, berating and threatening behaviour; and bullying and harassment is deliberate or hurtful behaviour (DH, 1999), which includes racism, homophobia, religious discrimination, sarcasm and name calling, ignoring someone (not being inclusive), and can be verbal, written or physical, or more increasingly in this day and age via mobile phone texts and emails. There are physical and behavioural indicators of abuse that may be exhibited, which the coach should look out for, and the typical signs are:

- unexplained bruising or injuries
- sexually explicit language or actions
- sudden changes in behaviour
- something a child has said
- a change is observed over a long period of time.

(Lester, 2003)

These signs may not constitute abuse and there may be other behavioural changes which the coach should be aware of, or even a cluster of signs. It is not the coach's responsibility to decide whether or not a child is being abused, but it is the coach's responsibility to act if there are any concerns. If a child discloses:

- Stay calm – ensure that the child is safe and feels safe.
- Show and tell the child that you are taking what they say seriously.
- Reassure the child and stress that they are not to blame.
- Be honest – explain that you will have to tell someone to help stop the abuse.
- Make a note of what the child said as soon as possible after the disclosure.
- Involve parents where appropriate.
- Maintain confidentiality – only tell others if it will protect the child.
- Follow guidelines laid down by either GBoS, Local Authority or SportsCoachUK.

(Lester, 2003; SSP, 2004)

Never:

- rush into actions that may be inappropriate
- make promises that you cannot keep
- take sole responsibility – consult someone (the person in charge or someone you can trust) so you can begin to protect the child and gain support for yourself
- go directly to the parents of the disclosing child.

The coach should also consider when coaching children that there are other instances when they should be aware of how they conduct themselves, and not put themselves in a position in which accusations could be levelled against them. This means not being in changing rooms alone with children, not taking a child to their home, ensuring that adults do not travel alone in cars with children, ensuring rooming arrangements are such that no adult is sharing with a child, and ensuring they do not touch a child inappropriately, even to the extent of putting an arm around the child, which could be misconstrued by someone who is standing a distance away.

The coach should not feel isolated when working with children and understand that there are individuals and organizations who they can voice their concerns to. In terms of reporting suspected cases of child abuse, the coach can report to:

- a senior coach
- the Welfare Officer of the club or organization
- GBoS child protection unit
- Childline
- Social Services
- the NSPCC
- the police.

A body now exists funded by the NSPCC and Sport England which was formed in 2001, called the Child Protection in Sport Unit (CPSU) and whose mission is to safeguard the welfare of children and young people under 18 in sport, promote their well-being and end child abuse by helping sports and other agencies to:

- Recognize their responsibility to protect children and young people in their care.
- Develop strategies and standards to protect children and young people.
- Identify and respond to adults who are a threat to children and young people.
- Develop child protection knowledge and skills among staff and volunteers.

(NSPCC, 2009, p. 1)

COACHING CHILDREN

Coaches play a major role in ensuring that children have a positive experience in sport, and at the same time in enhancing and developing their social skills. One of the major factors to consider when coaching children is self-esteem. A child's self-esteem is the value or worth attached to the self-description. Research supports the notion that a child's self-worth, or self-perceived physical capabilities, is a significant factor in their sport-related behaviour (Duda, 1987). If the child attaches low value to themselves, then it is likely that they will be low in self-confidence and consequently drop out of sport.

Self-esteem is influenced by parents, peers, teachers and coaches. The way the child feels or perceives his or her self is critical to a child's ability to function effectively as an individual (Pemberton and McSwegin, 1993). Sport plays a major role in the development of self-esteem (self-concept) in a young person, and research has generally found that sport improves self-concept in children (Horn, 1992). If young performers feel good about themselves after completing a task successfully, then their self-esteem is likely to increase. Coaches therefore should ensure that young performers have successful experiences (Hagger, 2003).

There are many reasons why children participate in sport, such as for fun, enjoyment, learning new skills, to be with friends and parental influence, and the two most important things when running a coaching session for children are fun and safety. Participating in sport also helps to improve their physical fitness and their technical, team and social skills. Alternatively, children may give up sport for a number of reasons, e.g. weather, cost of participating and buying equipment, not being selected for a team, poor coaching or lack of organization at a club.

To offset a potential negative experience of sport the coach should set a good example and ensure the experiences that children have in coaching sessions is positive. This is achieved by the coach being enthusiastic, being a good role model, setting realistic objectives, being organized, giving praise, pitching sessions at the right level for the ability and by being equitable. When coaching mixed groups it is important to understand the differences between boys and girls, therefore the coach should consider the following general points:

- Boys are usually more competitive and boisterous.
- Girls are keen to please and apply themselves well in practice.
- Girls physically and mentally mature on average two years ahead of boys.
- Boys develop physical strength earlier than girls – therefore the coach has to make considerations when coaching mixed gender groups.
- Girls often lack self-confidence and need more encouragement.
- Due to earlier puberty changes, girls can become more emotional.

(Adapted from Hagger, 2003)

Furthermore, the coach needs to consider the stage of motor learning that the child is at because it will affect their learning – their stage depends on physical growth and neurophysiological development. Before puberty there are relatively few gender differences (McMorris, 2004; McMorris and Hale, 2006), but children's limb lengths can be disproportionate in relation to their body, which may affect skill execution and movement (Hagger, 2003).

However, there are variations in gender with the onset of puberty, which can have a major effect on the way males and females perform skills. Generally, boys' strength improves, girls' less so. Boys and girls increase muscle mass, boys more so (McMorris, 2004) and this can impact upon agility, coordination and balance. The coach needs to understand that the young performer may go through a stage of being uncoordinated during puberty, and will have to be patient and adapt practices to account for the physical and motor development needs of the individual.

When planning a coaching session there are other considerations that the coach needs to acknowledge, which are different to those when coaching adults. The coach should:

- Take a register.
- Have prior knowledge of medical information and/or special needs.
- Provide parental consent forms.
- Have a programme of activities inclusive of dates and venues.
- Have ground rules appropriate for children, e.g. disciplined behaviour, parents dropping off and picking up children, late parent picking up procedure, parent contact details.
- Understand the Code of Conduct for Sports Coaches and the ethical responsibilities of the coach's relationship with children.
- Consider ability levels.
- Use appropriate levels of intended intensity of training for the group.
- Use appropriate clothing for activity (indoors or outdoors).
- Use appropriate environment for the session (indoors or outdoors).

When delivering a session for children the coach will also have to consider any adaptations that need to be made to the coaching session in order to provide effective and safe sessions for children. These can be outlined as follows:

- Modify equipment or size of equipment to allow safe practice.
- Modify the rules, or change the rules to allow safe practice.
- Develop fun-focused activities.
- Adapt training methods to meet the needs of the group – do not over-train.
- Group children according to ability and physical size.
- Modify length of time allocated to training and competition.
- Provide variety in sessions.
- Keep competition in perspective.
- Set appropriate and realistic targets.
- Use clear demonstrations coupled with simple explanations.
- Give enough time for practice.
- Be patient and correct errors one at a time.
- Coach bite-size, simple movements first.
- Use small sided games – let them play.
- Use question and answer technique to test understanding and engage with the child.

(Adapted from Hagger, 2003; Robinson, 2006a, 2006b)

Young children can suffer from heat stress and dehydration and be affected by cold far more than adults, and there are signs that the coach should look out for and then take action if needed during practices and competition.

Signs:

- change in colour and pallor

- tiredness and lethargy
- change in attitude
- lack of concentration
- breakdown in skill.

Action:

- Take them inside if it is too cold.
- If too hot, rehydrate in the shade.
- Change to lighter intensity activities.
- Use simple focused tasks.
- Use fun tasks.

(Adapted from Hagger, 2003)

THE LONG TERM ATHLETE DEVELOPMENT PROGRAMME

In making some general observations of sporting systems in the UK and around the world (mostly in swimming), Gordon (2008) has highlighted a range of issues that impact upon effective development of athletes. Gordon identified that: young athletes under-train and over-compete; inappropriate training programmes are implemented for young athletes; coaches' knowledge of critical periods in an athlete's development was limited; and that many of the best coaches were encouraged to work at the elite level when they could have better served at the developmental level imparting their knowledge and experience.

Considering this, it would not be unreasonable to suggest that a coherent, structured and methodical young athlete development pathway is required in order to facilitate the effective growth and development of the performer from their early years through to retirement. During the 1960s and early 70s, based on information regarding training methods and training programmes introduced in the Soviet Bloc countries (Siff, 2003), it became apparent that long-term planning of sports performance was a significant factor in achievement of international sporting success.

Studies done by the Soviets and East Germans underlined the importance of annual and quadrennial planning and training programmes (Gambetta, 2008) and this greatly contributed to the theory of training – especially with the introduction of the concept of multiple periodization (Balyi, 1990). With knowledge gained from the Soviet Bloc countries, the athletic performance development model, known as the Long Term Athlete Development (LTAD) model was developed by Istvan Balyi. The LTAD was originally developed in 1990 as a four-stage model and further evolved from five stages in 2001 to six stages in 2004.

The LTAD is one of a "number of approaches that focus on key, common principles of individual development, which has helped sports organizations to consider good practice in long-term planning for young athletes" (Stafford, 2005). The basic principles behind the LTAD model are:

- A training, competition and recovery programme based on biological and not chronological age.
- An athlete centred and coach driven model accounting for human development.
- A model underpinned by sports science.
- Provide periodized plans that are individualized to account for athlete needs.

- Provide a pathway for optimizing potential and lifelong participation in sport.

(Hagger, 2003; Stafford, 2005)

Balyi and Hamilton (2004) realized that athletes specialized in different sports at different stages so they classified sports into either early or late specialization sports. Early specialization refers to the fact that some sports, such as gymnastics, require early sport-specific specialization in training, and late specialization sports, such as athletics and team sports, require a generalized approach to early training. In late specialization sports, the emphasis of training should be on the development of general, fundamental motor and technical-tactical skills (Balyi, 2002).

A four-stage model was proposed to account for the early specialization sports, which includes training to train, training to compete, training to win and retirement or retaining. To account for late specialization a five-stage model was proposed which includes FUNdamentals. In 2004 the late specialization sport five-stage model was extended to a six stages, which includes learning to train (Balyi and Hamliton, 2004). The core components of the six stages which have been reduced for brevity are as follows (for more detailed information on all of these stages see Balyi, 2002; Hagger, 2003 and Stafford, 2005):

- FUNdamentals: 6–8 years for girls and 6–9 years for boys – the building of general motor skills which create a foundation in an individual's subsequent development in sport and physical activity.
- Learning to Train: 8–11 years for girls and 9–12 years for boys – learning all fundamental sports skills; the major learning stage for basic general sports skills.
- Training to Train: 11–14 years for girls and 12–15 years for boys – strengthening development of sport-specific skills and the introduction of tactical and performance development.
- Training to Compete: 14–17 years for girls and 15–18 years for boys – refining skills and performance and the structuring of training to replicate competition, together with the integration of sports science.
- Training to Win: 17+ years for girls and 18+ years for boys – maximization of skills, tactical and performance development.
- Retaining: lifelong participation – adjustment to retirement; retain athletes for coaching, officiating or performance as a veteran.

(Balyi, 2002; Hagger, 2003; Stafford, 2005)

COACHING THE DISABLED PERFORMER

Participation in sport activities for people with disabilities continues to gain in popularity (Ferrara and Peterson, 2000). The Paralympic Games and Special Olympics are now being attended by more and more athletes and are being provided with significantly more media coverage and reporting than ever before. Moreover, Paralympians are moving towards parity in many areas that have been easily accessible to their able-bodied counter-parts for many years, e.g. sports science support.

A landmark judgement was made in May 2008 when the Court of Arbitration for Sport overturned an original ruling by the International Association of Athletics Federations (IAAF), that Oscar Pistorius, double leg amputee and world record holder in the 100, 200 and 400 m could not compete for a place on South Africa's Olympic team using his carbon fibre prosthetic limbs. The reason for the original ban was that the IAAF ruled that his prosthetic "blades" provided him with a mechanical advantage over able-bodied athletes, but the Court of Arbitration for Sport ruled that they were not convinced that the device gave Pistorius an overall "metabolic advantage" and ruled that he should be allowed to compete in the 2008 Beijing Olympics.

Unfortunately, Pistorius did not make the qualifying time in Lucerne, Switzerland for a place on the South African Olympic Team to compete in the 2008 Olympic Games. However, Natalie de Toit became the first female leg amputee to swim in an able-bodied Olympics, when she took part in the 10 km open water event at Beijing and finished in 16th place out of 25 contenders.

The English Federation of Disability Sport (EFDS) has produced an activity based model called the Inclusion Spectrum that can help explain the contribution of including of disabled participants into sports sessions, and focuses on ability rather than disability (Kerr, 2003). The Inclusion Spectrum (EFDS, 2003) proposes five approaches to the delivery of sport programmes, such as:

■ Open activities – everyone does the same thing (deaf archers doing the same training as hearing archers).

■ Modified activities – everyone does the same task, but with a change to the rules (allowing a bounce of the ball in sit-down volleyball).

■ Parallel activities – everyone participates in the same activity, but different groups participate in different ways (in football the rules and size of the playing area for each group would differ).

■ Disability sport activities – non-disabled participate in an activity that has a disability sport focus; reverse integration (for example, boccia, where able-bodied athletes can compete alongside disabled athletes).

■ Separate activity – disabled participants play separately in an activity that has been adapted to their needs (for example, zone hockey where hockey sticks have been adapted to suit the needs of wheelchair use).

(Adapted from Kerr, 2003)

There have been barriers to participation for the disabled athlete in terms of viewing themselves as athletes; acceptance by team mates, coaches and officials; access to quality coaching; coaches having insufficient knowledge in disability sports and access to sports science and medicine (DePauw and Gavron, 2005). However, many of these barriers have now been broken down and the disabled athlete is gaining access to a range of support services and systems that have long been available to the able-bodied athlete.

Some ex-elite disabled athletes have even moved into coaching themselves. For example, Tanni Grey-Thomson, the Great Britain wheelchair athlete who has won 11 gold, four silver and one bronze in the Paralympic Games and has held 30 world records, is coaching wheelchair athletes, on top of writing and TV presenting.

It is true that the requirements of athletes with a disability can be in some cases be different to those of others (Kelly, 2007), however coaches should not view this as a convenient barrier to them working with disabled athletes. Coaching disabled athletes is not a difficult task if you accept each participant as an individual. The coach should however be aware of each person's abilities and the level at which the athlete is capable of movement or skill execution. There are further considerations that the coach should account for when coaching disabled athletes:

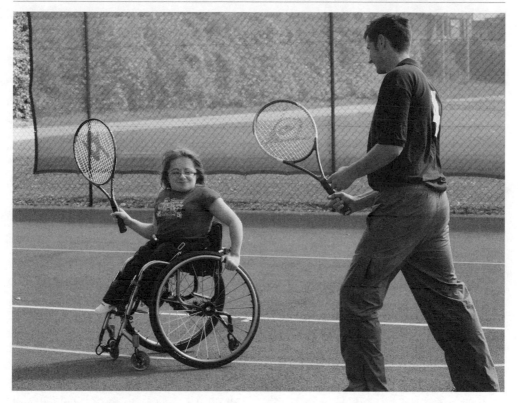

Photo 18.1 A coach working with a disabled performer.

- Physical capability – the athlete may have difficulties with movement, a low level of fitness, tire more quickly, experience balance and coordination problems.
- Cognitive – the athletes may find it hard to concentrate for long periods, and the coach may have to reinforce coaching points because some delay in transfer of learning may exist.
- Social – the athlete may be resistant to change, have difficulty with transition and routines, and may be easily frustrated and afraid to fail.
- Safety – extra precautions may have to be taken for emergency evacuation and access.

(Kerr, 2003)

However, Kelly (2003, p. 22) does suggest that "it is recognized that young people who have a congenital disability will have experienced fewer opportunities to develop physical skills, motor and movement literacy, and the apparent lack of functional ability in some can mask significant motor potential; equally those with an acquired ability can often both quickly and successfully transfer aspects of their previous motor learning to a wide range of sport activities". The message really is that the coach should have an open mind as to the capabilities of disabled athletes, and be prepared to adapt their coaching to suit the individual needs of the athletes. There are a range of considerations and approaches that the coach might want to be aware of when coaching disabled performers:

- Listen to the athlete.
- Seek out other disabled athletes in the event and ask their advice.
- Recruit able-bodied coaches as well as disabled coaches.
- Read texts and publications to gain an insight into disabled sport.
- Contact the disabled sport organization to find out further information.
- Film practices and competition for immediate visual feedback.
- Consult with technical experts about adaptive equipment.
- Investigate the disabled athlete's motivational methods to train and compete.
- Become familiar with the rules or rule changes.
- Experiment with new techniques.
- Keep a log or diary for the coach and athlete to determine trends that may enhance or hinder performance.

(Adapted from Gailey, 2004 and Kerr, 2003)

The coach may also have to consider his or her communication and coaching style and adapt the way they plan. In essence, the coach will have to challenge and adapt their beliefs in terms of the coaching process.

SUMMARY

Coaches should make themselves familiar with child protection issues, and at the same time not put themselves in a position where allegations could be levelled against them. There are different categories of abuse, such as neglect, physical, sexual and emotional abuse, and bullying and harassment. The CPSU exists as an organization whose mission is to safeguard the welfare of children and young people under 18 years in sport, to promote their well-being and end child abuse. Coaches play a major role in ensuring that children have a positive experience in sport, and at the same time in enhancing and developing their social skills.

Sport plays a major role in developing the self-esteem or self-concept of a young person and there are a number of reasons why children participate in sport such as, for fun, enjoyment, learning new skills, to be with friends, and parental influence, and the two most important things when running a coaching session for children are fun and safety.

The coach needs to consider the stage of motor learning that the child is at because it will affect their learning – their stage depends on physical growth and neurophysiological development. Gender variations are evident with the onset of puberty. The LTAD is one of a number of approaches that focus on key, common principles of individual development, and has helped sports organizations to consider good practice in long-term planning for young athletes (Stafford, 2005). The LTAD model describes six stages through which the athlete transits in their sporting career: FUNdamental, Learning to Train, Training to Train, Training to Compete, Training to Win and Retaining.

Participation in sport activities for people with disabilities continues to gain in popularity, and disabled athletes are now afforded the same access to a range of services and systems that have long been available to the able-bodied athlete. The Inclusion Spectrum is a model developed by the English Disability Sport Federation that can contribute to the understanding of the inclusion of disabled participants into sports sessions, and focuses on ability rather than disability.

SEMINAR OR DISCUSSION QUESTIONS

1. What practical coaching strategies can the coach employ in their coaching sessions to ensure that the young performer has a positive experience of sport?
2. In a sport of your choice, how would you adapt your coaching to suit the needs of the disabled performer participating in that sport?

KEY TERMS AND DEFINITIONS

- Bullying and harassment – deliberate or hurtful behaviour.
- Disability sport activities – non-disabled performers participate in an activity that has a disability sport focus.
- Emotional abuse – constant criticism, sarcasm and name calling.
- Inclusion Spectrum – model which helps explain the contribution of including disabled participants into sports sessions.
- Long Term Athlete Development Programme (LTAD) – lifelong participation in sport model.
- Modified activities – everyone does the same task, but with a change to the rules.
- Neglect – exposing children to undue cold, heat or unnecessary risk or harm.
- Open activities – everyone does the same thing.
- Parallel activities – everyone participates in the same activity, but different groups participate in different ways.
- Physical abuse – over-training or weight suppression.
- Self-esteem – value or worth attached to the description of oneself.
- Separate activity – disabled participants play separately.
- Sexual abuse – when adults or children (male or female) use children to meet their own sexual needs.

WEB LINKS

British Paralympic Association – www.paralympics.org.uk
Child Protection in Sport Unit – www.nspcc.org.uk/cpsu
Coaching disabled performers – www.efds.net
Long Term Athlete Development (LTAD) – www.sportdevelopment.org.uk

FURTHER READING

Child Protection in Sport Unit (2003). *Standards for Safeguarding and Protecting Children in Sport*. Sport England and NSPCC, London.
David, P. (2004). *Human Rights in Youth Sport: A Critical Review of Children's Rights in Competitive Sport*. Taylor & Francis, London.
DePauw, K. P. and Gavron, S. J. (1995). *Disability and Sport*. Human Kinetics, Champaign, IL.
Hagger, M (2003). *Coaching Young Performers*. Coachwise/SportsCoachUK, Leeds.

Kerr, A. and Stafford, I. (2003). *Coaching Disabled Performers*. Coachwise/SportsCoachUK, Leeds.
Lester, G. (2003). *Protecting Children: A Guide for Sportspeople*. Coachwise/SportsCoachUK, Leeds.
Stafford, I. (2005). *Coaching for Long-term Athlete Development: To Improve Participation and Performance in Sport*. Coachwise/SportsCoachUK, Leeds.

Chapter 18

Lifestyle management

CHAPTER OBJECTIVES

- Explain lifestyle management.
- Highlight the issues surrounding drugs and supplementations.

LIFESTYLE MANAGEMENT

Life in the twenty-first century is becoming increasingly busier and trying to maintain a balance between different and competing life areas can be problematic, even for the most organized person. The life areas that impact upon an individual's time are, for example, family, friends, financial pressures, relationships, education, socializing, work and rest. For the athlete it becomes more complicated as they have to fit in training, competition and travelling into an often already busy lifestyle.

Sport can be an important part of an athlete's life regardless of whether they are a recreational or elite athlete, and this can equally apply to the coach. However, sport is only part of an athlete's or coach's life, no matter how big a part it plays (Gastin, 2004) and it is a question of maintaining the right balance in comparison to other demands that compete for their time. The coach can play a major role in ensuring that the athlete does have a balanced lifestyle, by ensuring that they eat properly, do not over-train and get appropriate rest periods between training and competition.

While there seems to be support systems in place for the athletes to address maintenance of a balanced lifestyle, as of yet there are limited support systems in place for the coach. However, many of the concepts that are applied to the athlete can also be applied to the coach, and it could be suggested that having a mentoring system is an effective method of ensuring that coaches maintain a balanced lifestyle.

The way an athlete makes decisions about lifestyle factors is called lifestyle management (Earle, 2003) and encompasses two major principles: provision of a firm basis on which to train and compete, and managing risk, such as injury prevention and illness (Gastin, 2004).

Sports organizations have realized the importance of educating athletes in maintaining a balanced lifestyle, and of preparing the athlete for life after competition. UK Sport have implemented a Performance Lifestyle initiative, which is an "individualized support service specifically designed to help each athlete create the unique environment necessary for their success" (UK Sport, 2008b). Support services include time management, financial advice, dealing with the media, sponsorship and advertising, careers and employment advice and educational guidance. Governing Bodies of Sport for athletics, cricket and field hockey employ lifestyle advisers to support their athletes, and some UK universities offer support services to athletes in order to educate them about managing their lifestyles effectively.

Gastin (2004) suggests a number of different approaches that can be used to address the issue of lifestyle management, such as constructing a lifestyle profile, understanding how to make choices regarding competing demands on time, acknowledging that there are periods in an athlete's life that are stressful, and addressing the issue of maintaining balance in life areas.

The lifestyle profile (Gastin, 2004) assesses the current lifestyle of an individual and can identify current strengths and weaknesses in life areas, e.g. education and finances. If weaknesses are identified then a goal setting programme can be implemented to achieve lifestyle equilibrium. Choices have to be made on a daily basis, and there are times when an athlete or coach will argue that they have too much to do and not enough time to do it. If this is the case, then maybe it is time to do something about it. For the young athlete, school and sport quickly compete in deciding on a career and/or staying in education, and in whether to socialize or try and support themselves and raise a family (Gastin, 2004), and choices have to be made prioritizing which is important.

Tom Daley the 15-year GB diver who participated in the 2008 Beijing Olympic Games has had to make sacrifices in life areas so that he maintains a focus on his training and competition schedule: "Saturdays is the only time I get to see my mates, but I also have to spend time with family, one week I'll go to the cinema with my friends, the next day I'll have a day out with my family – I have had to make sacrifices with my schoolmates and not go to parties as I have had to rest at home or go training" (Daley, 2008 cited in Barkham, 2008).

Different sports have different demands in terms of training and competition and athletes are involved in an array of training and competition cycles, which will mean that there will be periods when allocation of time to other life areas other than sport will be limited. The rowing training regime of Sir Steven Redgrave the GB five-time Olympic gold medallist meant that he was training virtually every day, and he has even admitted to training on Christmas Day (Redgrave, 2008).

Debbie Flood, the GB Olympic rower who won silver at both the 2004 Athens and 2008 Beijing Olympic Games trains six hours a day, seven days a week, with just three weeks off a year after summer. "We don't have weekends, lie-ins, we train in the sun, wind, rain and hail and it's not easy" (Flood, 2008 cited in Kelso, 2008). These are just two examples of elite athletes who have dedicated a significant amount of time to their sport, maybe at the expense of other life areas.

A well constructed and implemented season plan or training programme that includes extensive and maximal training loads is fine as long as there are sufficient transition recovery periods that allow the athlete time to rest and allocate to other life areas. However, athletes can be single minded in their approach to training and competition. Sir Steven Redgrave openly admits he hated training but it was a means to an end for him. Being single minded and making sacrifices is fine, but it should not be to the detriment of one's health, relationships, career or education because there is a life after sport. An athlete's life can be stressful, especially during heavy training periods and upcoming competitions, and this could be coupled with being away from family and pressure from work. If these happen to coincide then there is potential for added pressure.

Gastin's (2004) lifestyle stress planner highlights four main areas (sport, work, study and life) and encourages athletes to look at all these areas and identify and record stress points that may impact upon performance. If an area is identified as being stressful early then the coach and athlete can make adjustments to the training programme in order to minimize the potential impact it could have on the athlete.

For example, an athlete who also serves in the armed forces may have an important competition coming up during a major military exercise or deployment. This would be highlighted as a stressful time for the athlete, and the coach could either adjust the training load or negotiate with the military the possibility of the athlete being exempted from the exercise or deployment, which would result in potentially less stress for the athlete.

DRUGS AND SUPPLEMENTATION

Unfortunately, drugs permeate all levels of sport, whether it is the Olympic athlete or recreational bodybuilder taking steroids or the recreational runner taking analgesics to combat the pain of shin splints in order to carry on running. The coach can play a significant role in educating the athlete in the dangers of taking performance enhancing and indeed recreational and over-the-counter drugs. The coach has a moral duty to ensure that their athletes are not tempted to take performance enhancing drugs, and certainly to not be complicit in aiding and abetting in illegal drug use.

The use of illicit compounds has been around since Ancient Greek times, when athletes were known to have used special diets and stimulating potions (Wadler and Hainline, 1989) and in the nineteenth century strychnine, caffeine, cocaine and alcohol were used by endurance athletes (Propkop, 1970). A number of initiatives have been implemented since 1928 when the International Athletics Federation was the first organization to ban the use of doping. However, restrictions were ineffective as no tests were performed.

Most international federations began testing in the 1970s, but already anabolic steroids were becoming widespread. During the 1990s increased drug detection rates were evidenced, which correlated with the decrease in world record performance in some strength related sports at the time (UK Sport, 2008c). The International Olympic Committee (IOC) set up the World Anti-Doping Agency (WADA) in 1999 as the international independent organization created to promote, coordinate and monitor the fight against doping in sport in all forms. The IOC has since established a Court of Arbitration for Sport, introduced out-of-competition testing and funded early research into doping trends and detection methods (Rogge, 2007).

Athletes over the years have used a range of drugs and methods in order to shave that one-hundredth of a second, lift that extra ten kilos or jump that one centimetre higher. These drugs and methods include the use of steroids, stimulants, diuretics, peptide hormones and analogues, blood doping, beta-blockers, narcotic analgesics, alcohol and beta$_2$ agonists. Also, a range of herbal and nutritional supplements have been tried, however many of these are unlicensed and not as strictly controlled as medicines. The biggest risk is cross contamination of supplements as the ingredients "are not what they say is in the tin" and if buying from the internet the athlete cannot be sure of what they are getting.

Drug testing unfortunately is now commonplace before, during and after major sporting events. The IOC and WADA planned to conduct 4,500 tests in Beijing (2008 Olympics), an increase on the 3,667 carried out four years earlier at Athens and a 90 per cent increase on the 2000 Sydney Olympic games (Barclay, 2008). The tests were carried out in the training or holding camps, in the Olympic Village or anywhere that WADA wanted to do them. WADA also indicated that any athlete who tested positive during the 2008 Beijing Olympics would not be going to London in 2012 (Juck and Elder, 2008). For the period April 2008–April 2009 UK Sport carried out a total of 7,545 drug tests as part of the national anti-doping programme, resulting in 32 confirmed anti-doping rule violations being added to the Drugs Results Database, together with 20 possible anti-doping rule violations (UK Sport, 2009a).

UK Sport is also making plans to establish a national anti-doping agency, under the banner of United Kingdom Anti-Doping (UKAD). UKAD will take on the testing and education programmes currently carried out by UK Sport, and will have significant new powers that link to law enforcement agencies. The management of doping cases will also be centralized (UK Sport, 2009b).

Anti-doping rules are based on the principle of strict liability and therefore supplements are taken at an athlete's risk and it is their personal responsibility. However, a new battlefront has emerged in the form of gene doping, which is defined as "the non-therapeutic use of cells, genetic elements, or the modulation of gene expression, having the capacity to improve athletic performance" (WADA, 2005, p. 3). Gene doping is the illegal counterpart of gene therapy. Gene therapy is available to treat muscle wasting disorders, whereby the patient is given a synthetic gene which can last for years, producing high amounts of naturally occurring muscle building hormones (Barber and Fiorino, 2008). The synthetic gene chemicals are indistinguishable from their natural counterparts and are produced locally in the infected tissue of the muscle, so nothing unusual enters the bloodstream, meaning anti-doping officials will have nothing to detect in a blood or urine test. This form of doping has the effect of synthetically producing muscle mass using a method that is undetectable.

Speaking at the 3rd WADA Gene Doping Symposium, Arne Ljungqvist (2008) suggested that "most experts do not think that gene transfer is being misused by athletes yet, but there is a growing level of interest for the potential of gene doping, and scientists who are working on genetic cures have already been approached by sports persons enquiring about the use of gene doping as a performance enhancement tool in sport". In order to combat this threat WADA is already funding research to understand the effects of gene doping on the human body and looking at early methods of detection (UK Sport, 2008f).

SUMMARY

Sport can be an important part of an athlete's life regardless of whether they are a recreational or elite athlete and this can equally apply to the coach. The coach can play a major role in ensuring that the athlete has a balanced lifestyle, by ensuring that they eat properly, do not over-train and get appropriate rest periods between training and competition. The way an athlete makes decisions about lifestyle factors is called lifestyle management (Earle, 2003).

Lifestyle management encompasses two major principles: provision of a firm basis on which to train and compete, and managing risk such as injury prevention and illness (Gastin, 2004). A number of different approaches can be used to address the issue of lifestyle management, such as using a lifestyle profile, making choices, acknowledging the question of balance and assessing lifestyle stress.

Unfortunately, drugs permeate all levels of sport and the use of performance enhancing drugs can be traced back to Ancient Greece. The International Athletics Federation was the first organization to ban the use of doping. However, use of performance enhancing drugs has become an issue for sport organizations, in terms of trying to keep one step ahead of the cheats. During the 1990s increased drug detection rates were evidenced, which correlated with a decrease in world record performances in some strength related sports at the time (UK

Sport, 2008c). A new battlefront has emerged in the form of gene doping which is defined as the "non-therapeutic use of cells, genetic elements, or the modulation of gene expressions, having the capacity to improve athletic performance" (WADA, 2005, p. 3) and WADA are funding research to combat this new threat.

SEMINAR OR DISCUSSION QUESTIONS

1. Identify the major lifestyle factors, allocate time spent on those each week and consider whether or not you have a balanced lifestyle.
2. Debate whether or not you think an athlete should be free to compete in the Olympics after completing a drugs ban.

KEY TERMS AND DEFINITIONS

- Gene doping – the non-therapeutic use of cells, genetic elements or the modulation of gene expression that has the capacity to improve athletic performance.
- Lifestyle balance – lifestyle factors in equilibrium.
- Lifestyle management – way in which the athlete makes decisions about lifestyle factors.
- Lifestyle profile – assesses the current lifestyle of an individual.
- Lifestyle stress planner – process used to identify potential periods of stress in an athlete's life.
- Performance enhancing drugs – various substances, chemical agents or procedures designed to provide an advantage in athletic performance.

WEB LINKS

Performance lifestyle – www.eis2win.co.uk
Professional and Athletes Life Skills – www.ucsport.net and follow link to PALS
World Anti Doping Agency – www.wada-ama.org

FURTHER READING

Butcher, R., Hong, F. and Schneider, A. (2006). *Doping in Sport*. Routledge, London.
Earle, C. (2003). Lifestyle management for young athletes. *Faster, Higher, Stronger*, 20, 16–17.
Gastin, P. (2004). Lifestyle management. *Faster, Higher, Stronger*, 23, 18–22.
Miah, A. (2004). *Genetically Modified Athletes*. Routledge, London.
Mottram, D. R. (2005). *Drugs in Sport*. Routledge, London.
Tamburrini, C. and Tannsjo, T. (2005). *Genetic Technology and Sport*. Routledge, London.

Chapter 19

Talent programmes

CHAPTER OBJECTIVES

- Explain the process of talent identification.
- Explain the process of talent transfer.

TALENT IDENTIFICATION

Kluka (2005) suggests that there is little doubt that coaches, athletes and those involved in sport search for answers as to what makes a champion athlete, how performance success can be predicted and what role sports science and technology play in creating an environment conducive to performance excellence.

The aim of talent detection and identification is to provide an "accurate prediction of those individuals who have the potential to compete at world-class levels" (Wolstencroft, 2002, p. 25). Talent is defined as "an aptitude or ability in one direction, above the normal average" (McCurdy, 2006 cited in Pluim, 2006, p. 6). Many coaches at some stage of their career will be involved in talent identification, whether it is on a micro level (e.g. recommending that a junior player at a club has the talent to move up into the senior squad), or on a more focused level (e.g. the soccer scout travelling the country talent spotting young players to sign up for a club on professional terms).

Talent identification is not a new concept. In the late 1960s and early 1970s Eastern European and Soviet Bloc countries established scientific methods to identify potential high performance athletes, with scientists masterminding the selection processes and procedures, and advising the coaches on which young people had the required abilities for sport (Crespo and McInerney, 2006). This policy produced dramatic results in the Munich (1972), Montreal (1976), Moscow (1980) and Los Angeles (1984) Olympic Games, for which several medallists were scientifically selected, especially from the former East Germany (Bompa, 1994).

In 1976, 80 per cent of Bulgarian medallists were the result of a thorough talent identification process (Bompa, 1994). Also, in 1976 Romanian scientists implemented a talent identification process for rowing, in preparation for the 1980 Moscow Olympic Games, with the result of one gold, two silver and two bronze medals. At the 1984 Los Angeles Olympic games they achieved five golds and at the 1988 Seoul Olympic games nine medals (Bompa, 1999).

Different countries have different approaches towards talent identification, and it can make all the difference to a country's performance in elite sports (Ainsworth, 2004). Kluka (2005) suggests that there are three general categories of talent identification systems: the systematic governmental system used by former Soviet Bloc countries and China, which is a state sponsored system; the systematic non-governmental system which is characterized by a developmental structure, which reinforces talent moving through well structured age group programmes; and a non-systematic system, which is a random, fragmented and unstructured system that has no particular approach.

Prior to the 2008 Beijing Olympic Games China implemented an intensive talent identification and training programme similar to that of the former Eastern Soviet Bloc. This programme was initiated in 2001 and called Project 119. The programme targeted selected sports that China was traditionally weak in, and was named after the number of gold medals offered in those track and field, swimming and other water based sports, such as rowing (Jones, 2008). A huge injection of money was poured into sport, sports technology and technical and coaching expertise to facilitate this project and the whole country was scoured by scouts looking for young athletes who might be able to compete in sports otherwise unknown in China. The result was that China headed up the medals table, with an astonishing 51 gold, 21 silver and 28 bronze medals.

Sport organizations in the UK are utilizing a hybrid systematic approach and integrating sports science to identify and tap into the talent pool ready for the 2012 London Olympics. However, unlike the Soviet and Eastern Bloc system, the UK system is not fully interwoven into the political system, although the UK government does provide some funding for sport on top of National Lottery funding. Moreover, for political purposes the British government would have no hesitation in basking in the reflected glory of successful athletes. This was more than evident when British Prime Minister Gordon Brown welcomed the medal winning GB athletes back from the 2008 Beijing Olympic games on the tarmac at Heathrow airport in August 2008.

Bompa (1994, 1999) identifies two different methods of talent identification. The natural approach assumes the athlete goes through the normal channels of playing sport, i.e. school, wishes of parents or peer pressure (Bompa, 1999). However, Crespo and McInerney (2006) argue that this model relies in part on the coincidence that the performer may begin to participate in sport, which means the process is not effectively utilized. The scientific approach is where the coach selects youngsters who have a proven ability and scientific testing is conducted in order to direct the individual to a specific sport (Bompa, 1999). However, Crespo and McInerney (2006) again argue that scientific models do not allow for the whole picture, in that there are other intangible aspects as well social influences that impact upon the development of talented performers.

Ainsworth (2004), Bompa (1994, 1999) and Wolstencroft (2002) propose that characteristics such as specific biological profiles, outstanding biomotor abilities, strong psychological traits and a high level of commitment should provide the foundation for talent identification criteria. However, if an individual has a handicap or lacks the necessary abilities, excessive training cannot overcome this lack of natural ability.

Whether or not it is agreed that using scientific methods for talent identification and selection is appropriate and effective, there are distinct advantages in using scientific criteria for talent identification:

- It reduces the time required to reach high performance by selecting individuals who are gifted in a sport.
- It eliminates a high volume of work, energy and talent on the part of the coach.
- The coach can maximize his or her training effectiveness by developing performers who have the potential aptitude and ability to become high class performers.

- It increases competitiveness in the talent pool and the number of athletes aiming at and aspiring to high performance.
- It increases athletes' self-confidence.
- It utilizes a pool of motivated sports scientists.

(Adapted from Bompa, 1994, 1999)

In early 2007 UK Sport, in partnership with the English Institute of Sport (EIS), implemented an initiative called Sporting Giants (UK Sport, 2007). A nationwide search for particularly tall athletes between the ages of 16 and 25 was conducted, with the aim of identifying potential Olympians in the sports of handball, volleyball and rowing. In February 2008, after a comprehensive and rigorous testing procedure, which included testing physical and psychological attributes, the ability to acquire sport-specific skills, game intelligence, arm span and vertical reach, UK Sport and the EIS announced that 34 rowers, 11 handball players and seven volleyball players had been successfully integrated into British squads (UK Sport, 2008d).

In June 2008, UK Sport and the EIS, together with major soccer authorities, challenged over 1,000 released academy players to switch their talents to targeted Olympic sports. The aim of the programme, called Pitch2Podium, is to provide young soccer players (aged 18–22 years) who have not yet secured a professional soccer contract with a unique opportunity to succeed in an alternative Olympic sport (UK Sport, 2008e).

TALENT TRANSFER

"Talent transfer is one area of talent identification that is shown to have merit in fast tracking talent, which involves elite athletes, and retired or nearly retired elite athletes switching sports and being provided with structured second chance opportunities to trial in a similar sport" (Yates *et al.*, 2007, p. 12). With appropriate coaching, support services and environments, these "ready made" athletes can be fast tracked into an Olympic sport.

Some highly publicized examples of talent transfer include Shelley Rudman, who won a silver medal in the 2006 winter Olympics in the bob skeleton less than four years after transferring from the 400 m track hurdles. Rebecca Romero, the 2004 Olympic rowing silver medallist, switched to track cycling and won the National Championships in less than a year. She went on to win silver in her first international World Cup event and a gold medal in track cycling at the 2008 Beijing Olympic Games. Alisa Camplin, the former Australian gymnast, won gold in aerial skiing at the 2002 winter Olympics after only four years on skis – she had never been on skis until the age of 22.

In the UK it was announced in October 2007 by the EIS that a handpicked group of artistic gymnasts, tumblers and gym acrobatic performers had made their first tentative steps on the road to potential success in the diving pool at the 2012 London Olympics, thanks to the UK Sport and EIS Talent Transfer Programme (EIS, 2007).

SUMMARY

The aim of talent identification is to provide "an accurate prediction of those individuals who have the potential to compete at world-class levels" (Wolstencroft, 2002). Talent identification is not a new concept. In the late 1960s and early 1970s Eastern European and Soviet Bloc countries established scientific methods to identify potential high class athletes, with scientists directing the selection procedures and advising coaches on which youngsters had the required abilities for sport. Throughout the 1960s, 1970s and 1980s the Soviet Bloc's system of talent identification reaped rewards in terms of medal hauls in a range of sports at the Olympics. UK Sport, in partnership with the EIS, has implemented an initiative called Sporting Giants, with the aim of identifying potential Olympians in the sports of handball, volleyball and rowing. Two methods of talent identification – natural and scientific – have been proposed, and three categories of talent identification system have also been identified – the systematic governmental, non-systematic governmental and non-systematic approaches.

Characteristics such as specific biological profiles, outstanding biomotor abilities, strong psychological traits and a high level of commitment should form the basis of criteria for talent identification, and the sports scientist plays a key role in identifying these characteristics. Talent transfer is one area of talent identification that is shown to have merit in fast tracking talent, which involves elite athletes, and retired or nearly retired elite athletes, switching sports and being provided with structured second chance opportunities to trial in another sport (Yates et al., 2007). With appropriate coaching, support services and environments, these "ready made" athletes could be fast tracked into an Olympic sport.

SEMINAR OR DISCUSSION QUESTIONS

1. In a sport of your choice identify criteria which could be used for talent identification.
2. Identify which sports might be suitable for an athlete to transfer his or her talents between.

KEY TERMS AND DEFINITIONS

- Non-systematic – a random system, with no particular approach.
- Systematic governmental system – government sponsored talent identification system.
- Systematic non-governmental system – not state sponsored, focuses more on a development structure.
- Talent identification – a system used to provide an accurate prediction of those individuals who have the potential to compete at world-class levels.
- Talent transfer – a pathway or system that involves elite athletes, and retired or nearly retired elite athletes, switching sports and being provided with structured second chance opportunities to trial in a similar sport.

WEB LINKS

Talent identification and talent transfer – www.uksport.gov.uk
Talent identification and talent transfer – www.eis2win.co.uk
Talent identification and talent transfer – www.ausport.gov.au

FURTHER READING

Bompa, T. (1994). *Periodization: Theory and Methodology of Training*. Human Kinetics. Champaign, IL.
Bompa, T. (1999). *Periodization: Theory and Methodology of Training* (4th edn). Human Kinetics. Champaign, IL.
Brown, J. (2001). *Sports Talent: How to Identify and Develop Outstanding Athletes*. Human Kinetics, Champaign, IL.
Yates, I., Dunman, N. and Warr, C. (2007). Unearthing London 2012 talent: The latest in talent transfer. *Coaching Edge*, 9, 12–13.

Appendix 1

Health and safety checklist

Venue:

Date:

Telephone location:

First aid location:

Emergency telephone numbers:

Local hospital:

Is my insurance in date?	
Have I completed a risk assessment?	
Do I have a copy of NOPs or EOPs?	
Do I have players' medical details?	
Do I have parents' telephone numbers (if working with children)?	
Have I completed a facility check?	
Is the equipment I am using serviceable?	
Is my first aid kit fully stocked?	
Do I have sufficient accident report forms?	
Have I constructed a session plan that meets the needs of the individual and group?	
Have I accounted for players' personal safety (injuries and jewellery, etc.)?	
Have I ensured that the players have the correct kit?	

Any further comments:

Appendix 2

Risk assessment form

Facility:	Group:	Date:	Completed by:	Next review date:
Hazard	Who is affected (coach, players or public)?	Risk rating (high, medium or low)	Action	Adjusted risk rating (high, medium, low)

Foundations of Sports Coaching, Routledge © Paul E. Robinson, 2010

Appendix 3

Accident report form

Name and location of facility:

Full name of lead/head/
senior coach:

Full name of injured person:

Full address of injured person:

Age of injured person:

Date of accident:

Time of accident:

Nature of injury, including
location on the body:

Nature of any post injury effects:

Full details of the accident. How
and where accident happened,
what activity was being
conducted:

Witness(es) name(s) and
address(es):

Immediate action taken:

Police called   Ambulance called   Parents called
YES/NO   YES/NO   YES/NO

Facility manager informed   Facility accident book completed
YES/NO   YES/NO

Details of first aid given:

Do the procedures in place require review? (if yes then please state):

Appendix 4

Practice needs analysis

Criteria	Practice needs
Name of player(s):	
Previous experience/ability:	
Individual needs:	
Aims and objectives:	
Size of group:	
Male/Female:	
Location:	
Session timings:	
Equipment needs:	
Medical information – to be kept in a secure location:	
Health and safety issues:	
Availability of support staff/ parents/helpers:	
Comments:	

Appendix 5

Session plan

Date: 2/2/2002

Session number: 2

Group size: 16

Session objective: Moving to and away with the ball, and opposite movement to clear space

Ability of group: Intermediate club level – female

Resources: Balls, bibs, cones, whistle, coach board and assistant coach

Skill and timings	Content and organization
1800–1815 Warm-up	Jog, static stretches (predominantly working on lower limb and back stretches) Use of ladders and hurdles for footwork exercises to link in with moving to and away with the ball
1815–1830 Introductory exercise	Re-visit passing exercise that focused on first touch last week
1830–1850 Skills	Moving to and away with the ball: 1. Pre-scan 2. Preparation phase (hands on stick, on toes and in balance) 3. Receive early and soft hands on first touch 4. Differentiation – moving away to the left and right

Player

Ball

| 1850–1920
Tactical theme or
modified game | Opposite movement to clear space:
1. Pre-scan
2. When to lead, where to lead, types of lead
3. Re-lead if need be
4. Early shot on goal
5. Add in defenders to increase pressure |

P1 & P2 make leads

Pass

Pass

| 1920–1930
Cool-down | Jog, and static stretches to focus on calves, quads, hamstrings and lower back muscles |

Appendix 6

Evaluation

Date: 4/2/2002   **Coach name:** A. Coach

Session number: 2   **Support staff:** Assistant Coach

What went well:

My coaching style was appropriate to the needs of the group. The progression from moving to and away with the ball, to the opposite movement, to clear space practice went well. My health and safety brief was also good, and I ensured that the players had an exit route on the second exercise. Generally, the players responded well to the feedback and to the reason why the exercise was delivered at this key point in the season (an observation was made from the previous game that movement was limited in forward play). There was an exception to this in that a disagreement arose between the coach and two senior players.

What did not go so well:

My communication of some of the coaching points was not so good. I feel that I did not explain the first exercise as well as I should have done, which resulted in two players not knowing which side of the cone they were meant to be coming out from. This resulted in the two players getting frustrated, which subsequently resulted in a mild disagreement with the coach about why this particular exercise was being conducted.

How the session could be improved:

I should have explained the first exercise better, which would have limited any conflict arising. The disagreement distracted me from providing effective feedback at key points during this exercise, and impacted upon the needs of the rest of the group. While I was trying to explain the reasons behind the exercise for the two players who were questioning me, I could have suggested that we discuss this at a more appropriate time at the end of the session, which would have allowed me to account for all the needs of the group.

Action to be taken for next session:

Reflect during this next week upon how I communicate technique and strategies. Fully explain the purpose of an exercise, and put it fully in the context of a game. Speak to the two senior players to ask them if there is any way I can communicate better in order to account for their needs.

Appendix 7

Block planner

Performer's name:	Individual or group:	Date:	Block planner number:
Summer Salt	Trampolinist	7/2/2002	2

Session	Skill/Technique	Tactics/Performance	Fitness
Overall aims and objectives	Development of four somersaults	Incorporate into a ten-jump routine Six previous jumps were practised during the previous block planning cycle	• Flexibility • Plyometrics • Trampoline-specific conditioning
One	Back somersault – tucked • Take-off • Mid-phase • Landing	Seven-jump routine	• Flexibility • Plyometrics • Trampoline-specific conditioning
Two	Back somersault – piked • Take-off • Mid-phase • Landing	Eight-jump routine	• Flexibility
Three	Front somersault – half twist • Take-off • Mid-phase • Landing	Nine-jump routine	• Plyometrics
Four	Crash dive • Take-off • Mid-phase • Landing	Ten-jump routine	• Flexibility • Plyometrics • Trampoline-specific conditioning
Evaluation and look forward to next cycle	All techniques completed All ten techniques from previous block plan and this plan will be reinforced over the next block planning cycle	Ten-jump routine executed in good form Will reinforce the whole ten-jump routine in preparation for the next competition phase in two weeks	All fitness components completed and integrated into skill technique and ten-jump routine Will increase intensity of fitness components in preparation for next competition phase

Appendix 8

Performance requirement analysis for boxing

Performer's name: Walter Waite

Weight division: Welterweight

Cycle: Annual/Biennial/Quadrennial: Annual

Coach's name: B. Glove

Period: 2000 – 2001

Physical	Agility, balance, explosive strength, flexibility, muscular endurance, muscular power, reactions Include aerobic endurance for road runs
Technical	Ring craft – footwork and punching Punch bag and speed bag work

Tactical	Three styles:
	  1. Front foot boxing
	  2. Back foot boxing
	  3. Combination of both
	Southpaw and orthodox → account for opponents' styles also

Psychological	Concentration, control the controllables, focus, goal setting, mental toughness, motivation to train
Weight management	Reduction in weight from welterweight (69 kgs boxing weight) to light welterweight (64 kgs boxing weight)
Sparring partners	Identification of three sparring partners to account for three differing styles

University men's field hockey season plan

Macro	One				Two			Three			Four		
Month	Jul.	Aug.	Sept.	Oct.	Nov.	Dec.	Jan.	Feb.	Mar.	Apr.	May	Jun.	
Week (micro)	4 11 17 25	1 8 15 22 29	5 12 19 26	3 10 17 24 31	7 14 21 28	5 12 19 26	2 9 16 23 30	6 13 20 27	6 13 20 27	3 10 17 24 1	8 15 22 29	5 12 19 26	
Training phases	RP2	GPP	SPP	CP1			RP3	CP2		RP1			
Meso	1A	1B	2	3	4	5	6	7	8	9	10	11	
Competition	Fitness	Fitness and technical	Pre Pre Pre Pre L / L L L L	L L L L L	L L L L	Rest and light aerobic work		L L L L L & & & & & C C C C C	L L L L	Light aerobic work – fitness plans provided to players for fitness maintenance			
Intensity 1–5	2 2 3	3 4 4 4 4	4 4 5	5 5 4 4 3	4 4 5	5 5 3 3 2	3 3 4 5 5	5 4 4 4 4	4 3 4	2 2 2 2	2 2 2 2 2	2 2 2	
Peaking		*	*		*			*					
Testing	T	T						T					
Component	Aerobic anaerobic and multi-directional	Multi-directional. SAQ. Plyometrics. Technical.	Technical and tactical training. One session per week			Maintain fitness		Technical and tactical work. Maintain and manipulate volume and intensity		Summer sports			
Goals	Fitness goals. Team and individual goals	Develop skills, new techniques and tactics	Set pieces; attack and defence strategies. Development and reinforcement of team patterns and tactics. Reinforcement of core skills and techniques. Continued reinforcement of new skills and techniques			Review and evaluate team and individual goals				Participation in summer sports to rest and recuperate			
Psychological	Short-/medium-/long-term goal setting	Mental imagery, concentration and arousal regulation	Mental imagery, concentration and arousal regulation			Goal review		Mental imagery and focusing techniques		Season review and goal evaluation			

Source: Adapted from Galvin and Ledger (1998) and Robinson (2005)

Appendix 10

Dietary analysis form

Name:

Include fluids	Monday	Tuesday	Wednesday	Thursday	Friday	Saturday	Sunday
Breakfast							
Mid-morning							
Lunch							
Mid-afternoon							
Dinner							
Evening							
Other extras							

Appendix 11

Fitness profile

Name:		Age:	Position/Event:
Fitness component			**Rating**
Aerobic endurance			1 2 3 4 5
Explosive power			1 2 3 4 5
Flexibility			1 2 3 4 5
Speed			1 2 3 4 5
Muscular endurance			1 2 3 4 5

Test	Time/Result									

Match statistics form

Opposition:	Date:
Team:	
Half-time score:	Full-time score:
Scorers:	
Goals won (open play):	Goals conceded (open play):
Short corners won:	Short corners lost:
Goals won (short corners):	Goal lost (short corners):
Long corners won:	Long corners lost:

Pass rate percentage: Success × 100 ÷ total = pass rate %

Glossary

Ability basic innate actions that underlie skilled performance.

Activist a person who likes learning by doing.

Acute injuries severe and intense injuries.

Adenosine tri-phosphate (ATP) an immediate energy system.

Aerobic system with oxygen.

Anaerobic system without oxygen.

Angular involving rotation around a central line or point.

Anthropometric related to the dimensions and weights of body segments.

Anticipation ability to have an expectation of or to predict upcoming events.

Arousal the physiological and/or cognitive readiness to act.

Balanced lifestyle having a lifestyle that is more or less equal in all parts and includes sport, family, friends, finances, education, etc.

Behavioural management theory a flexible and employee involved approach.

Block planner a scheme of work that highlights general aims and objectives over an extended six-week cycle.

Bullying and harassment deliberate or hurtful behaviour.

Cardiac contractions shortening of heart muscle initiated by electrical impulse.

Cardiac muscle forms the major part of the heart.

Centre of gravity point around which a body's weight is equally balanced.

Chronic injuries long-lasting injuries.

Classical management theory focuses on efficiency and includes bureaucratic, scientific and administrative management.

Coach educator a senior coach who delivers coach education courses to candidate coaches.

Coach licensing a policy that is being considered by SportsCoachUK, in order to regulate the coaching industry.

Coaching behaviour the behavioural responses exhibited by the coach in response to his or her performer's behaviour.

Coaching philosophy a moral set of beliefs that determine a coach's behaviour in a range of situations.

Coaching process a means by which coaching delivery is determined by the three core elements: Plan, Lead, Reflect.

Coaching style way in which the coach delivers their coaching session.

Code of conduct a set of values and principles which guides coaching practice.

Competition period period where the objective is to compete.

Concentration having the ability to attend to cues in the environment for prolonged periods of time.

Conflict resolution intervention by a coach or other person in disagreements between individuals.

Continuing professional development attending further learning opportunities that support the coach and coaching practice.

County Sports Partnership provides a single system of delivery of sport in the community.

Creatine phosphate secondary energy system; creatine phosphate is broken down to re-create ATP.

Decision making knowing what to do, when to do it and how to do it.

Demonstration provision of appropriate information for developing a memory template.

Department of Media, Culture and Sport government department responsible for government policy on sport.

Developmental coaching rapid skills learning and engagement with a sport-specific competition programme.

Differentiation changing the practice to account for the ability needs of the individual.

Digestion the breaking down of food.

Digitization a performance analysis process using digital technology.

Disability sport activities non-disabled performers participate in an activity that has a disability sport focus.

DOMS Delayed onset muscle soreness.

Dynamic Flex® warm-up and cool-down process, which incorporates multi-directional movement while stretching.

Dynamic stretching moving while stretching.

Emergency operating procedures a policy that provides information on fire, evacuation and emergency procedures.

Emotional abuse constant criticism, sarcasm and name calling.

Environmental injuries result of exercising or performing in extreme weather conditions.

Evaluation a process by which the coach highlights their strengths and weaknesses and how they could improve their coaching sessions.

External respiration exchange of gases between lungs and the blood.

Extrinsic motivation doing the activity for reward or praise factors.

Feedback meaningful information regarding skill execution provided from either an internal or external source.

Fitness component a specific demand of a sport (e.g. aerobic endurance).

Fitness testing process by which the coach can assess and monitor a performer's fitness levels.

Force push or pull; the product of mass and acceleration.

Foundation coaching coaching at the beginner or junior level.

Friction force acting on the area of contact between two surfaces in the opposite direction to the motion or impending motion.

Gene doping the non-therapeutic use of cells and genetic elements or the modulation of gene expression, having the capacity to improve athletic performance.

General motion motion inclusive of translation and rotation simultaneously.

General preparatory period general conditioning which is characterized by large quantities at low volume.

Goal an objective, aim of some action or level of performance.

Governing Body of Sport   a sport-specific organization that looks after the interests of that sport.

High performance coaching   coaching at the elite level.

Human relations management theory   provides a more human perspective towards management.

Human resource management   the effective management of people.

Imagery   ability to mentally re-create objects, persons, skills, experiences and situations while not physically being involved in those situations.

Impact injuries   result of direct contact with an opponent or piece of equipment.

Inclusion Spectrum   model which helps explain the contribution of including disabled participants into sports sessions.

Individualization   an individualized training programme.

Individualized training plans or programmes   a specific training programme tailored to the needs of the individual performer.

Inertia   tendency of a body to resist change in its state of motion.

Internal injuries   result of stresses on joints, ligaments, tendons or muscles.

Internal respiration   carriage of gases by the blood and the exchange of gases between blood and cells.

Intrinsic motivation   doing the activity for its own sake.

Kinematics   form, pattern, or sequencing of movement with respect to time.

Kinesiology   study of human movement.

Kinetics   study of the action of forces.

Learning   a relatively permanent change in performance.

Learning style   "the complex manner in which, and conditions under which, learners most efficiently and most effectively perceive, process, store and recall what they are attempting to learn" (James and Gardner, 1995, p. 20).

Lifestyle balance   lifestyle factors in equilibrium.

Lifestyle management   way in which athlete makes decisions about lifestyle.

Lifestyle profile   assesses the current lifestyle of an individual.

Lifestyle stress planner   process used to identify potential periods of stress.

Linear   along a line, straight or curved, with all parts of the body moving in the same direction at the same speed.

Long Term Athlete Development Programme   lifelong participation in sport model.

Long-term memory   holds information for long periods of time.

Macro cycle   long-term cycle.

Management theory   a principle idea that provides a framework with which to understand the processes that are involved in management.

Managing the coaching environment   maintaining group control of a practice.

Mass   quantity of matter contained in an object.

Mediator   someone who intervenes to settle a dispute.

Mentor   a senior coach who in developing a one-to-one relationship supports the development of another coach.

Meso cycle   medium-term cycle.

Micro cycle   short-term cycle.

Modified activities   everyone does the same task, but with a change to the rules.

Motivation   the direction and intensity of one's effort.

Multi-directional training   development of a range of biomotor skills such as agility, balance, coordination, quickness and speed.

Neglect   exposing children to undue cold, heat or unnecessary risk or harm.

Non-systematic   a random system, with no particular approach.

Non-verbal communication   body language.

Normal operating procedures   a policy which provides information on the day-to-day running of a facility.

Notational analysis   process used to gather objective data on the performance of athletes.

Observation   what to look for in a logical order.

Open activities   everyone does the same thing.

Over-use injuries   result of using a specific body part repetitively.

Parallel activities   everyone participates in the same activity, but different groups participate in different ways.

Part-continuous practice   each component is introduced in a continuous and progressive logical sequence so that they all gradually build up to form the whole technique.

Participation coaching   initiation into the sport and delivering basic skills plus accounting for the recreational and casual participant.

Part-progressive   each component is practised in isolation before being recombined and practised together.

Peaking   a process by which the performer reaches optimal physical performance.

Performance analysis   analysing individual, team or squad performance utilizing a range of methods.

Performance coaching   relatively intensive preparation and involvement in competition sport.

Performance enhancing drugs   various substances, chemical agents or procedures designed to provide an advantage in athletic performance.

Periodization   division of a programme into distinct training periods.

Physical abuse   over-training or weight suppression.

Practice needs analysis   a process used in order for the coach to gather information to identify and account for certain needs in the planning process.

Pragmatist   likes learning by trying.

Pre-conditioning   training to train.

Pre-cooling   a process that helps regulate the body's core temperature.

Pre-performance routine   a sequence of task-relevant thoughts, actions and procedures designed to provide an advantage in athletic performance.

Professional coach   one who is in paid full-time employment as a coach.

Projection speed   the magnitude of projection velocity.

Pulmonary ventilation   breathing.

Reaction time   the speed at which we make decisions.

Reactive behaviour   the coach's reaction to the team or performer.

Rectilinear   along a straight line.

Reflect   to review and evaluate coaching performance.

Reflector   likes learning by discussion.

Re-hydration   effective fluid replenishment.

Residual volume   air left in the lungs after each breath.

Risk assessment   a system that identifies items and situations that may cause accidental injuries or health problems.

SAQ®   Speed, Agility and Quickness   a concept that focuses on developing fundamental motor abilities.

Season plan long-term scheme of work covering either an annual, biennial or quadrennial cycle.

Selective attention ability to pick out relevant cues in the environment.

Self-confidence an individual's belief in their ability.

Self-esteem value or worth attached to the description of one's self.

Sensory store holds information for around 250 milliseconds.

Separate activity disabled participants play separately.

Sequential progression a progression of overload situations leading into tactical or game play.

Session plan an organized scheme of work that allows the coach to deliver, monitor and assess specific aims and objectives of practice.

Sexual abuse when adults or children (male or female) use children to meet their own sexual needs.

Short-term memory holds information for around 30 seconds.

Situation-specific or contingency theories suggest an interaction between the leader and the situation.

Skeleton bone struture that supports the body by giving it shape, and also provides attachment points for the muscles.

Skill the ability to bring about pre-determined results with maximum certainty, often with the minimum of outlay of time, energy or both.

Smooth muscle mostly found in layers and forms the muscle part of the digestive tract, the bladder, blood vessels and the skin.

Specific preparatory period period for specific skill and technical development prior to the start of the competition period.

Spontaneous behaviour initiated by the coach and is not in response to the behaviour of player(s).

SPORT a mnemonic for a set of principles to follow in order to train effectively.

Sports psychology a science in which the principles of psychology are applied in the sport and exercise setting.

State anxiety an emotional state that sees an elevation in physiological arousal.

Strength and conditioning a training method than concentrates on developing strength endurance.

Striated or skeletal muscle muscle attached to the skeleton.

SWOT analysis process to identify Strengths, Weaknesses, Opportunities or Threats.

Systematic governmental system government sponsored talent identification system.

Systematic non-governmental system not state sponsored talent identification system, focuses more on a development structure.

Talent identification a system used to provide an accurate prediction of those individuals who have the potential to compete at world-class levels.

Talent transfer a pathway or system that involves elite athletes, and retired or nearly retired elite athletes, switching sports and being provided with structured second chance opportunities to trial in another sport.

Tapering a reduction in training volume and an increase in training intensity.

Theorist likes learning facts.

Tidal volume resting air which moves in and out of the lungs with each breath.

Torque the rotary effect of force about an axis of rotation.

Total lung capacity the vital capacity plus the residual volume.

Training periods macro, meso and micro cycles.

Training plan an organized schedule of coaching over a period of time.

Training unit practice session.

Trait anxiety a personality variable.

Trait theory certain leaders have personality traits and personality characteristics that make them ideally suited for leadership.

Trajectory flight path of a projectile.

Transition recovery period recovery and having a break from training.

Type of practice a method of practice delivery.

United Kingdom Coaching Certificate an endorsement of coach education programmes across sports within the UK set against agreed criteria.

Universal behaviours the theory that successful leaders have certain universal behaviours.

Variability of practice use of different practice schedules to facilitate the learning process.

Verbal communication instruction.

Vital capacity largest amount of air that can be expelled from the lungs.

Volunteer an individual who helps others in sport through formal organizations such as clubs or governing bodies and is not paid to do so.

Warm-up decrement following a period of rest, sports performance will decrease temporarily.

Whole-part-whole the coach presents the whole practice, then the practice is broken down into its component parts before the whole is practised again.

References

Abraham, A. and Collins, D. (1998). Examining and extending research in coach development. *Quest*, 50, 59–79.

Active Schools (2008). Coaching for teachers. Online: www.eriding.net/resources/pe/030922_pe_active_schools.doc (accessed 14th October 2009).

Active Surrey (2008). Safeguarding and protecting children and young people in sport in Surrey: Play sport, Stay safe. Online: http://www.activesurrey.com/content-2087 (accessed 28 September 2009).

Ainsworth, C. (2004). Built to win. *New Scientist*, 2471, 50–3.

Allaby, M, (1999). A *Dictionary of Zoology*. Oxford University Press, Oxford.

AP (Associated Press) (2009). Central Michigan: Women's coach sued by ex-player. *Fox News* (Tuesday, 10 February), Associated Press.

Armstrong, M. (2006). A *Handbook of Human Resource Management Practice* (10th edn). Kogan Page Ltd, London.

ASC (Australian Sports Commission) (2008a). Coaching and officiating: Australia's national approach to coaching and officiating. Online: www.ausport.gov.au/participating/officials/education (accessed 14th October 2009).

ASC (2008b). Overview of mentoring. https://secure.ausport.gov.au/sports_official/mentoring/mentoring (accessed 28 September 2009).

ASEP (2008). About ASEP. Online: http://www.asep.com/about.cfm (accessed 28 September 2009).

Baechle, R and Earle, R. W. (2000). *Essentials of Strength Training and Conditioning*. Human Kinetics, Champaign, IL.

Bailey, S. (2007). *The Sports Source Book: A UK Directory of Sport*. ch. 9: Volunteering in sport. Coachwise/SportsCoachUK, Leeds.

Baker, A. (2006). *Coach Education Handbook*. England Hockey Development, Milton Keynes, England.

Baker, A. (2007). *Coach Education Handbook*. England Hockey Development, Milton Keynes, England.

Balyi, I. (1990). *Quadrennial and Double Quadrennial Planning of Athletic Training*. Canadian Coaches Association, Victoria, BC.

Balyi, I. (2002). Long-term athlete development: The system and solutions. *Faster, Higher, Stronger*, 14, 6–9.

Balyi, I. and Hamilton, A. (2004). *Long-term athlete development: Trainability in childhood and adolescence. Windows of opportunity, optimal trainability*. National Coaching Institute, and Advanced Training and Performance Ltd, Victoria, BC.

Bandura, A. (1977). Self-efficacy: Toward a unifying theory of behavioural change. *Psychological Review*, 84, 191–215.

Bandura, A. (1986). *Social Foundations of Thought and Action: A Social Cognitive Theory*. NJ, Prentice-Hall, Englewood Cliffs.

Barber, D. (2008). Football Association historian. Telephone communication (4 February).

Barber, P. and Fiorino, M. E. (2008). Potential new gene therapy strategy for muscle wasting diseases. *Medical News Today* (11 March). MediLexicon International Ltd.

Barclay, C. (2008). Olympics: New drugs testing for athletes. *The New Zealand Herald* (24 July). APN Holdings NZ Ltd.

Barkham, P. (2008). Making a splash. *Guardian* (3rd March). Guardian News and Media Ltd.

Barnett, T. (2009). Encyclopedia of Management | Management Thought. Online: http://www.enotes.com/management-encyclopedia/management-thought/print (accessed 27 November 2009).

Barron, J. and Gjerde, K. P. (1996). Who adopts Total Quality Management (TQM) theory: an empirical test. *Journal of Economics and Management Strategy*, 5(1), 69–106.

Bartlett, R. (1997). *Introduction to Sports Biomechanics*. Routledge, London.

Bartlett, R. (1999). *Sports Biomechanics*. Routledge, London.

Bartlett, R., Gratton, C. and Rolf, C. (2006). *Encyclopaedia of International Sports Studies*. Taylor & Francis, London.

Beashel , P. and Taylor, J. (1997). *The World of Sport Examined*. Thomas Nelson and Sons, Ontario.

Billat, V. L. (2001). Interval training for performance: A scientific and empirical practice. Special recommendations for middle and long distance running. Part 1: Interval training. *Sports Medicine*, 31(1), 13–31.

Bleak, J. L. and Frederick, C. M. (1998). Superstitious behaviour in sport; Levels of effectiveness and determinants of use on three college sports. *Journal of Sport Behaviour*, 21, 1–15.

Bompa, T. (1994). *Periodization: Theory and Methodology of Training*. Human Kinetics. Champaign, IL.

Bompa, T. (1999). *Periodization: Theory and Methodology of Training* (4th edn). Human Kinetics. Champaign, IL.

Boocock, S. (2007). Coaching children in the 21st century: Safe practice guidelines. *Coaching Edge*, 9, 20–1.

Borgers, M. (2008). Sports coaching structures in the Netherlands. Email communication (26 March).

Brackenridge, C. (2004). Silent voices: Consulting children in sport. Article based on a keynote speech to the annual conference of the Leisure Studies Association, Leeds Metropolitan University, July.

Brewer, C. (2005). *Strength and Conditioning for Games Players*. Coachwise/SportsCoachUK, Leeds.

British Council (2008). Career fact file: Sports Coach. Online: http://www.educationuk.org/pls/hot_bc/bc_subject_zone.page_pls_related_articles?x=186357801909&y=0&a=0&p_subj_id=2&p_subzone_id=22 (accessed 28 September 2009).

Brown, J. (2001). *Sports Talent: How to Identify and Develop Outstanding Athletes*. Human Kinetics, Champaign, IL.

Brown, L. E and Ferrigno, V. A. (2005). *Training for Speed, Agility and Quickness* (2nd edn). Human Kinetics, Champaign, IL.

Buhrmann, H. G., Brown, B. and Zaugg, M. K. (1982). Superstitious beliefs and behavior: A comparison of male and female basketball players. *Journal of Sport Behavior*, 5, 75–185.

Bull, S. J., Albinson, J. G. and Shambrook, J. (1996). *The Mental Game Plan: Getting Psyched for Sport*. Sports Dynamics, Eastbourne.

Burns, V. (2005). Could the brain of a monkey help to improve an athlete's performance? *Daily Telegraph* (29 November). Telegraph Media Group Ltd.

Burton, D. (1989). The impact of goal specificity and task complexity on basketball skill development. *Sport Psychologist*, 3, 34–47.

Butcher, R., Hong, F. and Schneider, A. (2006). *Doping in Sport*. Routledge, London.

CAC (Coaching Association Canada) (2005). Overview of Coaching Association of Canada. Online: http://www.coach.ca/eng/about_cac/overview.cfm (accessed 28 September 2009).

Caplan, G. and Adams, M. (2007). *Fitness Testing for Sport and Exercise*. BTEC National Sport, Butterworth-Heinneman, Oxford.

Carlson, A. (2008). Hydration for athletes. *Competitive Edge*, 4(1), 2.

Case, R. (1998). Leader member exchange theory and sport: Possible applications. *Journal of Sport Behaviour*, 21, 387–95.

Centre for Sport and Law (2000). More coaches being sued. *Coaches Report*, 6(4).

Chambers, D. (1997). *Coaching: The Art and the Science*. Key Porter, Toronto.

Chelladurai, P. (1980). Leadership in sport organizations. *Canadian Journal of Applied Sport Psychology*, 5, 226–31.

Child Protection in Sport Unit (2003). *Standards for Safeguarding and Protecting Children in Sport*. Sport England and NSPCC, London.

Christina, R.W. and Corcos, D. M. (1988). *Coaches Guide to Teaching Sports Skills*. Human Kinetics, Champaign, IL.

Chu, D. A. (1998). *Jumping into Plyometrics*. Human Kinetics, Champaign, IL.

Clegg, C. (1995). *Exercise Physiology and Functional Anatomy*. Feltham Press, Hampshire.

Clubmark (2008). About Clubmark. Online: http://www.clubmark.org.uk/about/about-clubmark

Cochrane, D. J. (2003). Alternating hot and cold water immersion for athlete recovery: A review. *Physical Therapy in Sport*, 1(5), 26–32.

Cole, J. (2008). Hydration, re-hydration and hyponatremia. Online: www.sportsinjuryclinic.net/cybertherapist/general/heat_injury.php (accessed 14th October 2009).

Connor, S. (2000). Sharkskin swimsuits lead hi-tech bid for Olympic gold. *Independent* (17 March). International News and Media.

Continyou (2007). Strategy Guide: Advice for PE and sport strategy managers in local authorities. Online: http://www.continyou.org.uk/files/documents/documents/doc_249.pdf (accessed 14 October 2009).

Cook, M. (2007). Periodization theory: A refresher. *Coaching Edge*, 7, 10–11.

Costill, D. I., King, D. S., Thomas, R. and Hargreaves, M. (1985). Effects of reduced training on muscular power in swimmers. *Physician and Sports Medicine*, 13, 94–101.

Cowan, K. (2005). Left brain-right brain theory. Journal entry communication. Ithaca College, New York.

Cowan, N. (2001). The magical number 4 in short-term memory: A reconsideration of mental storage capacity. *Behavioral and Brain Sciences*, 24, 87–185.

Cox, R. H. (1998). *Sport Psychology: Concepts and Applications* (4th edn). Mc-Graw-Hill, New York.

Cox, R. H. (2007). *Sport Psychology: Concepts and Applications* (6th edn). Mc-Graw-Hill, New York.

CPSU (2001). Working with sport to keep children safe. Online: http://www.nspcc.org.uk/Inform/cpsu/AboutUs/AboutUs_wda60534.html (accessed 14th October 2009).

Crespo, M. and McInerney, P. (2006). Talent identification and talent in tennis. International Tennis Federation. *Coaching and Sport Science Review*, 39, 2.

Crisfield, P. (2003). *Analyzing your Coaching*. Coachwise/SportsCoachUK, Leeds.

Crisfield, P., Cabral, P. and Carpenter, F. (2003). *The Successful Coach: Guidelines for Coaching Practice* (3rd edn). Coachwise/SportsCoachUK, Leeds.

Cross, N. and Lyle, J. (1999). *The Coaching Process: Principles and Practice for Sport*. Butterworth-Heinneman, Oxford.

Cushion, C. J. (2006). Mentoring: Harnessing the power of experience. In R. Jones (ed.). *The Sports Coach as Educator: Reconceptualizing Sports Coaching*. Routledge, Oxford.

Cuskelly, G., Hoye, R. and Auld, C. (2006). *Working with Volunteers in Sport: Theory and Practice*. Routledge, London.

Daley, T. (2008). Cited in Barkham, P. (2008). Making a splash. *Guardian* (3rd March). Guardian News and Media Ltd.

David, P. (2004). *Human Rights in Youth Sport: A Critical Review of Children's Rights in Competitive Sport*. Taylor & Francis, London.

Davis, R. J., Bull, C. R., Roscoe, J. V. and Roscoe, D. A. (1995). *Physical Education and the Study of Sport*. Moseby, London.

Dawson, T. (1993). *Principles and Practice of Modern Management* (ch. 10). Hodder and Stoughton, Kent.

DCMS (Department for Culture, Media and Sport) (2002). *The Coaching Task Force–Final Report*. Sport and Recreation Division of Department for Culture, Media and Sport. UK Government, England.

DePauw, K. P. and Gavron, S. J. (1995). *Disability and Sport*. Human Kinetics, Champaign, IL.

DePauw, K. P, and Gavron, S. J. (2005). *Disability Sport* (2nd edn). Human Kinetics, Champaign, IL.

Detling, N. (2008). Negative Motivation. Online: http://www.HeadStrongConsulting.com/newsletter.asp?title=Negative%20Motivation (accessed 28 September 2009).

DH (Department of Health) (1999). *Working Together to Safeguard Children: A Guide to Inter-agency Working to Safeguard and Promote the Welfare of Children*. Department of Health, England.

Douge, B., Alexander, K., Davis, P. and Kidman, L. (1994). *Evaluation of the National Coach Accreditation Scheme*. Australian Coaching Council.

Drawer, S. (2006). Looking to the future: Technology in high-performance sport. *Coaching Edge*, 4, 26–7.

Driscoll, J. (2005). Reflections on learning styles. *Faster, Higher, Stronger*, 28, 12–13.

Duda, J. (1987). Towards a developmental theory of motivation in sport. *Journal of Sport Psychology*, 9, 130–45.

Duffy, P. (2009). Opening address. 4th UK Coaching Summit. Glasgow, Scotland. 28–9 April.

Dulaney, S. (2001). Ethics in coaching. *The Sport Journal*, 4(3), 3–5.

Dunn, R. Dunn, K. and Price, G. (1987). *Learning Styles Inventory*. Price Systems, Lawrence, KS.

Earle, C. (2003). Lifestyle management for young athletes. *Faster, Higher, Stronger*, 20, 16–17.

Easterbrook, J. A. (1959). The effect of emotion on cue utilization and the organization of behaviour. *Psychological Review*, 66, 183–201.

Edmondson, S. R (2005). Evaluating the effectiveness of a telepresence-enabled cognitive apprenticeship model of teacher professional development. Doctoral dissertation. Utah State University, UT.

EFDS (English Federation of Disability Sport) (2003). *Inclusion Spectrum*. Manchester Metropolitan University, Stoke-on-Trent, England.

EIS (English Institute of Sport) (2007). Diving into new talent. Online: http://www.uksport.gov.uk/news/diving_into_new_talent/ (accessed 28 September 2009).

England Hockey (2006). *England Hockey Level One Coach Award*. England Hockey, Milton Keynes, England.

English Sports Council (1996). *A Summary of the Major Findings from a Sports Council Survey into the Voluntary Sector*. English Sports Council, London.

Ericsson, K. A. and Smith, J. (1991). *Towards a General Theory of Expertise; Prospects and Limits*. Cambridge University Press, Cambridge.

Eston, R. and Peters, D. (1999). Effects of cold water immersion on the symptoms of exercise-induced muscle damage. *Journal of Sports Science*, 17(3), 231–8.

Eustice, C. and Eustice, R. (2006). Sport Injury Guide. The common type of sports injuries. Online: http://arthritis.about.com/od/sportsinjuryarthritis1 (accessed 28 September 2009).

Eysenck, M. W. and Calvo, M. G. (1992). Anxiety and performance: The processing efficiency theory. *Cognition and Emotion*, 6, 409–34.

Eysenck, M. W. and Keane, M. T. (2005). *Cognitive Psychology* (5th edn). Psychology Press, Hove.

Feltz, D. L. and Lirgg, C. D. (2001). Self efficacy beliefs of athletes, teams and coaches. In: R. N. Singer, H. A. Hausenblas and C. Janelle (eds). *Handbook of Sport Psychology* (2nd edn) (pp. 340–61). John Wiley & Sons, New York.

Ferrara, M. S. and Peterson, C. L. (2000). Injuries to athletes with disabilities: Identifying injury patterns. *Sports Medicine*, 30(2), 137–43.

Filby, W. C. D., Maynard, I. W. and Graydon, J. K. (1999). The effect of multiple goal strategies on performance outcomes. *The Sport Psychologist*, 1, 224–36.

Fitts, P. M. and Posner, M. I. (1967). *Human Performance*. Brooks/Cole, Belmont, CA.

Flood, D. (2008). Cited in Kelso, P. (2008). Flood aims to turn the tide for Britain on a sea of faith. *Guardian* (6 August). Guardian News and Media Ltd.

Foran, B. (2001). *High performance sports conditioning*. Human Kinetics, Champaign, IL.

Foxon, F. (2001). *Improving Practices and Skills*, Coachwise/SportsCoachUK, Leeds.

Franks, I. M. and Miller, G. (1986). Eye witness testimony in sport. *Journal of Sport Behaviour*, 9, 39–45.

Frederick, A. M. and Frederick, C. (2006). *Stretch to Win*. Coachwise/SportsCoachUK, Leeds.

FSA (Food Standards Agency), (2008). Fats and cholesterol. Online: http://www.eatwell.gov.uk/healthissues/healthyheart/cholesterol/ (accessed 28 September 2009).

Gailey, R. (2004). Coaching athletes with disabilities: A 12 step program. *The Orthotics and Prosthetics Edge*, April.

Galvin, B. (2003). *A Guide to Mentoring Sports Coaches*. Coachwise/SportsCoachUK, Leeds.

Galvin, B. and Ledger, P. (1998). *A Guide to Planning Coaching Programmes*. Coachwise/SportsCoachUK, Leeds.

Gambetta, V. (2008). *Periodization and the Systematic Sport Development Process*. Gambetta Sports Training.

Gardner, T. (1999). Coaching and the law of the land. *Faster, Higher, Stronger*, 6, 6–8.

Gastin, P. (2004). Lifestyle management. *Faster, Higher, Stronger*, 23, 18–22.

Geddes and Grossett (1995). *Brockhampton Reference: Dictionary of Calories*. Brockhampton Press, New Lanark, Scotland .

Ghaye, T. (2001). Reflection: Principles and practices. *Faster, Higher, Stronger*. 10, 9–11.

Goodbody, J. (2008). Building great teams. *Coaching Edge*, 10, 5.

Goode, S. and Magill, R. A. (1986). The contextual interference effects in learning three badminton serves. *Research Quarterly for Exercise and Sport*, 57, 308–14.

Gordon, D. (2009). *Coaching Science*. Learning Matters, Exeter.

Gordon, R. (2008). *A Shorter Guide to the Long Term Athlete Development Programme*. Amateur Swimming Association.

Green, A. (2003). *Implementing the Recommendations of the Coaching Task Force: The Community Sports Coach Scheme*. Briefing Note, August. Sport England.

Green, D. P., Whitehead, J. and Sugden, D. A. (1995). Practice variability and transfer of a racket skill. *Perceptual and Motor Skills*, 81, 1275–81.

Griggs, G. (2008). Outsiders inside: The use of sports coaches in primary schools. *Physical Education Matters*, Spring, 33–6.

Grimshaw, P., Lees, A., Fowler, N. and Burden, A. (2006). *Instant Notes in Sport and Exercise Biomechanics*. Routledge, London.

Groner, G. (2004). Stretching out? Online: http://www.biomech.com/full_article/?ArticleID=848&month=10&year=2004 (accessed 28 September 2009).

Grosso, M. R. (2006). Training theory: A primer on periodization. *The Coach*, 33, 25–33.

Gupta, S., Goswani., D., Sadhukhan, A. K., and Mathur, D. N. (1996). Comparative study of lactate removal in short term massage of extremities, active recovery and a passive recovery period after supramaximal exercise sessions. *International Journal of Sports Medicine*, 17, 106–10.

Hagerman, F. C. (1992). Energy metabolism and fuel utilization. *Medicine & Science in Sports & Exercise*, 24(9), 309–14.

Hagger, M. (2003). *Coaching Young Performers*. Coachwise/SportsCoachUK, Leeds.

Halsall, R. (2006). Widening Participation. *Learning and Teaching in Action*, 4(2), 3–6.

Hall, S. B. (2007). *Basic Biomechanics*. McGraw-Hill, London.

Hamill, J. and Knutzen, K. M. (1995). *Biomechanical Basis of Human Movement*. Williams and Wilkins, London.

Hanin, Y. L. (1992). Social psychology and sport: Communication processes in top performance teams. *Sport Science Review*, 1(2), 13–28.

Hardman, A. E. and Stensel, D. J. (2003). *Physical Activity and Health: The Evidence Explained*. Routledge, London.

Hardy, L. and Fazey, J. (1987). The inverted-u hypothesis: A catastrophe for sport psychology? Paper presented at the Annual Conference of the North American Society for the Psychology of Sport and Physical Activity. Vancouver.

Hardy, C. A. and Mawer, M. (1999). *Learning and Teaching in Physical Education*. Routledge, London

Hardy, L., Beattie, S. and Woodman, T. (2007). Anxiety-induced performance catastrophes: Investigating effort required as an asymmetry factor. *British Journal of Psychology*, 98(1), 15–31.

Harter, S. (1978). Effectance motivation reconsidered. Towards a developmental model. *Human Development*, 21, 34–64.

Haskin, D. (2003). The mentoring process. *Faster, Higher, Stronger*, 18, 10–11.

Hay, J. G. and Reid, J. G. (1988). *Anatomy, Mechanics, and Human Motion*. Prentice-Hall, Englewood Cliffs, NJ.

Hay, J. G. (1993). *The Biomechanics of Sports Techniques* (4th edn). Prentice-Hall, Englewood Cliffs, NJ.

Heffner, C. L. (2001). Memory, intelligence, and states of mind (ch. 6 of Psychology 101). Online: http://allpsych.com/psychology101/memory.html (accessed 28 September 2009).

Henley, J. (2008). Yummy and . . . yuck. *Time Out*. (Sunday, 24 August). Time Out Group, London.

Herbert, R. D. and Gabriel, M. (2002). Effects of stretching before and after exercising on muscle soreness and risk of injury: A systematic review. *British Medical Journal*. 325, 468–70.

Herbert, V. H. and Subak-Sharpe (1995). *Total Nutrition: The Only Guide You'll Ever Need*. St Martins Press, New York.

Hickman, K. (2008). Hundred Years War: English Longbow. Online: http://militaryhistory.about.com/od/smallarms/p/englongbow.htm (accessed 28 September 2009).

Hinkson, J. (2001). *The Art of Team Coaching*. Warwick Publishing, Toronto.

Hodge, K. (2004). *The Complete Guide to Sport Motivation*. A & C Black. London.

Hodkinson, W. (2008). Grand Archery Association Historian. Telephone communication (21 February).

Honeybourne, J. (2006). *Acquiring Skill in Sport: An Introduction*. Routledge, London.

Honey, P. and Mumford, A. (2001). *The Learning Styles Helpers Guide*. Maidenhead, England.

Hong, Y. and Bartlett, R. (2008). *Routledge Handbook of Biomechanics and Human Movement Science*. Routledge, London.

Horizon (2006). *Winning Gold in 2012. Horizon Special*. BBC2, England.

Horn, T. S. (2008). *Advances in Sport Psychology* (3rd edn). Human Kinetics, Champaign, IL.

Houlihan, B. and White, A. (2002). *The Politics of Sports Development: Development of Sport or Development through Sport*. Routledge, London.

Hughes, M. (2005). From analysis to coaching – the need for objective feedback. Online: http://www.coachesinfo.com/index.php?option=com_content&view=article&id=305:analysis-to-coaching&catid=91:general-articles&Itemid=170 (accessed 28 September 2009).

Hughes, M. and Franks, I. (2004). *Notational Analysis of Sport: Systems for Better Coaching and Performance in Sport*. Routledge, London.

Hughes, A. and Reader, K. (2003). *Encyclopedia of Contemporary French Culture*. CRC Press, Florida.

Hull, C. L. (1943). *Principles of Behaviour*. Appleton-Century-Crofts, New York.

ICCE (International Council for Coach Education) (2008). About the ICCE. Online: http://www.icce.ws/about/index.htm (accessed 28 September 2009).

Ivy, J. L., Goforth, H. W. Jnr., Damon, B. M., McCauley, T. R., Parsons, E. C. and Price, T. B. (2002). Early post exercise muscle glycogen recovery is enhanced with a carbohydrate-protein supplement. *Journal of Applied Physiology*, 93(4), 1337–44.

James, W. B. and Gardner, D. L. (1995). Learning styles: Implications for distance learning. *New Directions for Adult and Continuing Education*, 67, 19–32.

Jarvis, M. (1999). *Sport Psychology*. Routledge, London.

Jones, G. (2008). China's Olympic plan to topple America. Online: http://www.thefirstpost.co.uk/45023, news-comment-news-politics,chinas-119-olympic-dreams (accessed 28 September 2009).

Jones, D. F., Housner, L. D. and Kornspan, A. (1997). Interactive decision making and behaviour of experienced and in-experienced basketball coaches during practice. *Journal of Recreation and Physical Education*, 16, 454–68.

Jones, R. l. (2006). *The Sports Coach as an Educator*. Routledge, London.

Juck, A. and Elder, L. (2008). IOC, WADA, USADA increasing tests in Beijing. *EME News*. Bratislava, Slovakia.

Kahneman, D. (1973). *Attention and Effort*. Prentice-Hall, Englewood Cliffs, NJ.

Kelly, K. (2007). Should you coach athletes with a disability differently? *Coaching Edge*, 8, 22–3.

Kelso, P. (2008). Flood aims to turn the tide for Britain on a sea of faith. *Guardian* (6 August). Guardian News and Media Ltd.

Kerr, A. and Stafford, I. (2003). *Coaching Disabled Performers*. Coachwise/SportsCoachUK, Leeds.

Kerry, D. (2008). Individualization. Great Britain Women's Head Coach. England Hockey. Telephone communication (14 April).

Ketcham, C. J. and Stelmach, G. E. (2004). *Technology for Adaptive Aging*. The National Academies Press, Washington, DC.

Kilgore, J. L and Touchberry, C. D. (2007). *Basic Fitness Testing: Field Tests for Sport and Fitness Professionals*. The Aasgaard Company Publishers, Texas.

Kluka, D. A. (2005). *Long-term Athlete Development: Systematic Talent Identification*. Department of Health, Physical Education and Sport Science, Kennesaw State University, USA.

Knapp, B. (1963). *Skill in Sport*. Routledge and Kegan Paul, London.

Knudson, D. and Kluka, D. A. (1997). The impact of vision and vision training in sport performance. *Journal of Physical Education Recreation and Dance*, 68, 8–17.

Kopelman, R. E., Prottas, D. J. and Davis, A. L. (2008). Douglas McGregor's Theory X and Y: Toward a construct-valid measure. *Journal of Managerial Issues*, Summer, 18, 393–408.

Kozoll, C. (1988). *Coaches' Guide to Time Management*. Springfield Books Limited, England.

Kriel, J. (2005). An outline of management (ch.1). In: G. Kriel, D. Singh, A. de Beer, H. Louw, J. Mouton, D. Rossouw, J. Berning and D. du Toit (eds). *Focus on Management: A Generic Approach*. Juta and Company Ltd, South Africa.

Lee, J. (2008). Ice baths for workout recovery. Online: http://speedendurance.com/2008/05/11/ice-baths-for-workout-recovery/ (accessed 28 September 2009).

Lee, M. (1993). *Coaching Children in Sport: Principles and Practice*. Taylor & Francis, London.

Leisure Jobs (2008). Online: http://www.leisurejobs.com

Lester, G. (2003). *Protecting Children: A Guide for Sportspeople*. Coachwise/SportsCoachUK, Leeds.

Levenhagen, D. L., Carr, C., Carlson, M .G., Maron, D. J., Borel, M. J. and Flakoll, P. J. (2002). Post exercise protein intake enhances whole-body and leg protein accretion in human. *Medicine & Science in Sport & Exercise*, 34(5), 828–37.

Lidor, R. and Singer, R. N. (2000). Teaching pre-performance routines to beginners. *The Journal of Physical Education, Recreation and Dance*, 71(7), 34–6.

Ljungqvist, A. (2008). WADA Gene doping Symposium calls for greater awareness: Strengthened action against potential gene transfer misuse in sport. WADA 3rd Gene Doping Symposium, St Petersburg, Russia, 11 June 2008.

Locke, E. A. and Latham, G. P. (1985). Application of goal setting to sport. *Journal of Sport & Exercise Psychology*, 7(3), 205–22.

Locke, E. A. and Latham, G. P. (1990). *A Theory of Goal Setting and Task Performance*. Prentice-Hall, Englewood Cliffs, NJ.

Lyle, J. (1999). Coaches' decision making. In: N. Cross and J. Lyle (eds). *The Coaching Process: Principles and Practice for Sport* (pp. 210–32). Butterworth-Heinneman, Oxford.

Lyle, J. (2002). *Sports Concepts: A Framework for Coaches' Behaviour*. Routledge, London.

Lyle, J. (2007). A review of the research evidence for the impact of coach education. *International of Sports Science and Coaching*, 1(1), 19–36.

McCurdy, D. (2006) cited in Pluim, B. (2006). Medical considerations when identifying talent. *Coaching and Sport Science Review*, 39, 6.

McKardle, W. D., Katch, F. I. and Katch, V. L. (2007). *Exercise Physiology: Energy, Nutrition and Human Performance* (6th edn). Lippincott Williams and Wilkins, London.

Mackenzie, B. (2008a). *101 Evaluation Tests – Train Smarter*. Electric Word, PLC.

Mackenzie, B. (2008b). Warm up and cool down. Online: http://www.brianmac.co.uk/warmup.htm (accessed 28 September 2009).

McLaughlin, D., Stamford, J. and White, D. (2006) *Instant Notes in Human Physiology*. Routledge, London.

McMorris, T. (2004). *Acquisition and Performance of Sports Skills*. Wiley & Sons, Chichester.

McMorris, T. and Hale, T. (2006). *Coaching Science: Theory into Practice*. Wiley & Sons, Chichester.

McNab, T. (1990). Chariots of Fire into the twenty-first century, *Coaching Focus*, 13, Spring, 2–5.

McNamara, C. (2008). Very brief history of management theories. Online: http://www.managementhelp.org/mgmnt/history.htm (accessed 28 September 2009).

McNamee, M. J. and Parry, S. J. (1998). *Ethics and Sport*, Routledge, London.

Magill, R. A. (1993). *Motor Learning: Concepts and Applications*. McGraw-Hill, New York.

Maglischo, E. W. (2003). *Swimming Fastest: A Comprehensive Guide to the Science of Swimming*. Human Kinetics, Champaign, IL.

Martens, R. (1987). *The Coaches' Guide to Sports Psychology*. Human Kinetics, Champaign, IL.

Martens, R. (2004). *Successful Coaching* (3rd edn). Human Kinetics, Champaign, IL.

Martens, R., Burton, D., Vealey, R., Bump, L. and Smith, D. (1990). The development of the Competitive State Anxiety Inventory-2 (CSAI-2). In: R. Martens, R. S. Vealey and D. Burton (eds). *Competitive Anxiety in Sport* (pp. 117–90). Human Kinetics, Champaign, IL.

Martinek, T. (1991). *Psycho-social Dynamics of Teaching Physical Education*. Wm. C. Brown. Dubuque, IA.

Matthews, J. (2008). Cricket courses in the UK. Email communication (23 January 2008).

Maughan, R. and Gleeson, M. (2004). *The Biochemical Basis of Sports Performance*. Oxford University Press, Oxford.

Maughan, R., Gleeson, M., and Greenhaff, P. L (1997). *Biochemistry of Exercise and Training*. Oxford University Press, Oxford.

Mechikoff, R. and Estes, S. (1998). *A History and Philosophy of Sport and Physical Education: From the Ancient Greeks to the Present* (2nd edn). Brown & Benchmark, Madison, WI.

Mehrabian, A. (1968). Communication without words. *Psychology Today*, 52–5.

Miah, A. (2004). *Genetically Modified Athletes*. Routledge, London.

Moran, G. T. (1996). *The Psychology of Concentration in Sport Performers: A Cognitive Analysis*. Psychology Press, Hove.

Moran, G. T. and McGlynn, G. H. (1997). *Cross Training for Sports*. Human Kinetics, Champaign, IL.

Morris, T., Spittle, M. and Watt, A. P. (2005). *Imagery in Sport*. Human Kinetics, Champaign, IL.

Mottram, D. R. (2005). *Drugs in Sport*. Routledge, London.

Nacson, J. and Schmidt, R. A. (1971). The activity set hypothesis for warm-up decrement. *Journal of Motor Behaviour*, 3, 1–15.

Nash, C. (2003). Development of a mentoring system within coaching practice. *Journal of Hospital, Leisure, Sport and Tourism Education*, 2(2), 39–47.

Nesti, M. (1992). Managing volunteers. *Recreation Management Facilities Fact File 1*. Sports Council, London.

Nettleton, J. A. (1995). *Omega-3 Fatty Acids and Health*. Springer Publishing, New York.

Newman, P. (2004). England send Grip to take a look at Johnson. *Independent* (Saturday 13 November 2004). Independent News and Media Ltd.

Nichols, J. G. (1984). Conceptions of ability and achievement motivation. In: R. Ames and C. Ames (eds). *Research on Motivation in Education: Student Motivation* (Vol. 1). Academic Press, New York.

Nideffer, R. (1976). Test of attentional and interpersonal style. *Journal of Personality and Social Psychology*, 34, 394–404.

Nideffer, R. M. and Sagal, M. (2001). Attention control in training. In: J. M. Williams, *Applied Sports Psychology; Personal Growth to Peak Performance* (4th edn), pp. 312–32. Mayfield Publishing Company, Mountain View, CA.

NHSCA (National High School Coaches Association) (2008). Online: http://www.nhsca.com (accessed 28 September 2009).

North, J. (2009). *The Coaching Workforce 2009–2016.* SportsCoachUK, Leeds.

NSPCC (National Society of Prevention of Cruelty to Children) (2007). Online: http://www.nspcc.org.uk/Inform/research/statistics/prevalence_and_incidence_of_child_abuse_and_neglect_wda48740.html (accessed 28 September 2009).

Nurse, N. (2003). Leading teams. *Faster, Higher, Stronger,* 19, 12–13.

Ophir, G., Amariglio, N., Jacob-Hirsch, J., Elkon, R., Rechavi, G. and Michaelson, D. M. (2005). Apolipoprotein E4 enhances brain inflammation by modulation of the NF-kappaB signaling cascade. *Neurobiology of Disease,* 20(3), 709–18.

Owen, M. (2003). Mentoring in context. *Faster, Higher, Stronger,* 18, 7–8.

Owens, L. and Stewart, C. (2004). *Understanding Athletes' Learning Styles.* International Society of Biomechanics in Sport, Coach Information Service.

Palastanga, N., Field, D. and Soames, R. (1998). *Anatomy and Human Movement: Structure and Function* (3rd edn). Butterworth-Heinemann, Oxford.

Pankhurst, A. (2007). *Planning and Periodization.* Coachwise/SportsCoachUK, Leeds.

Parfitt, C. G. and Hardy, L. (1987). Further evidence for the differential effects of competitive anxiety upon a number of cognitive and motor sub-components. *Journal of Sports Science,* 5, 62–72.

Parsons, J. (2005). *Hockey: Bridging the Gap Project.* Mentoring workshop, SportsCoachUK, Sussex County Sports Partnership, England.

Payne W., Reynolds M., Brown S. and Fleming A. (2002). *Sports Role Models and their Impact on Participation on Physical Activity: A Literature Review.* VicHealth and the University of Ballarat, Australia.

Pearson, A. (2004). *Dynamic Flexibility: Warming up on the Move.* A & C Black, London.

Pemberton, C. L. and McSwegin, P. J. (1993). Sedentary living: A health hazard. *Journal of Physical Education, Recreation and Dance,* 64(3), 27–31.

Plessinger, A. (2008). The effects of mental imagery on athletic performance. Online: http://www.vanderbilt.edu/AnS/psychology/health_psychology/mentalimagery.html (accessed 28 September 2009).

Plowman, S. A. and Smith, D. D. (2007). *Exercise Physiology for Health, Fitness and Performance.* Lippincott Williams & Wilkins, Philadelphia.

Pluim, B. (2006). Medical considerations when identifying talent. *Coaching and Sport Science Review,* 39, 6.

Poulton, E. C. (1950). Perceptual anticipation and reaction time. *The Quarterly Journal of Experimental Psychology,* 2(3), 99–112.

Poulton, E. C. (1957). On prediction in skilled movement. *Psychological Bulletin,* 54(6), 467–78.

Powers, S. K. and Howley, E. T. (1997). *Exercise Physiology: Theory and Application to Fitness and Performance* (3rd edn). WCB McGraw-Hill, New York.

Propkop, L. (1970). The struggle against doping and its history. *Journal of Sports Medicine and Physical Fitness,* 10(1), 45–8.

Quinn, E. 2007. Fast and slow twitch muscle fibres. Online: http://sportsmedicine.about.com/od/anatomyandphysiology/a/MuscleFiberType.htm (accessed 28 September 2009).

Quinn, E. (2008a). Eating after exercise – post exercise meal. Online: http://sportsmedicine.about.com/cs/nutrition/a/aa081403.htm (accessed 28 September 2009).

Quinn, E. (2008b). Interval training builds fitness fast: Vary your training intensity to boost your performance. Online: http://sportsmedicine.about.com/od/tipsandtricks/a/Intervals.htm (accessed 28 September 2009).

Quinn, E. (2008c). The warm up: How to warm up before exercise. Online: http://sportsmedicine.about.com/cs/injuryprevention/a/aa071001a.htm (accessed 28 September 2009).

Raab, M. (2003). Decision making in sports: Influence of complexity on implicit and explicit learning. *International Journal of Sport and Exercise Psychology,* 1, 310–37.

Raygor, A. L. and Wark, D. M. (1970). *Systems for Study.* McGraw-Hill, New York.

Redgrave, S. (2008). Me and my boat. Online: http://www.t5m.com/steve-redgrave/me-and-my-boat.html?fb=1&fb=1 (accessed 28 September 2009).

Reid, M., Crespo, M., Lay, B. and Berry, J. (2006). Skill acquisition in tennis: Research and current practice. *Journal of Science and Sports Medicine in Sport,* 10(1), 1–10.

Richfield, J. (2008). No swimming. *New Scientist*, 2638, 81.

Rikli, R. E. and Jones, C. J. (2001). *Senior Fitness Test Manual*. Human Kinetics, Champaign, IL.

Robergs, R. A. and Landwehr, R. (2002). The surprising history of the "HRmax = 220 age" equation. *Journal of Exercise Physiology Online*, 5(2), 1–10.

Robertson, K. (2002). *Observation, Analysis and Video*. Coachwise/SportsCoachUK, Leeds.

Robinson, P. E. (2005). *Season Planning for Hockey*. England Hockey Development, Milton Keynes, England.

Robinson, P. E. (2006a). *Level One Workshop Update:* England Hockey Development, England Hockey, Milton Keynes, England.

Robinson, P. E. (2006b). *Level Two Workshop Update*. England Hockey Development, England Hockey, Milton Keynes, England.

Robinson, P. E. (2006c). Selective attention. *Push*, 5(November), 48.

Rogge, J. (2007). Speech by Dr Jacques Rogges, President of the International Olympic Committee to the World Conference on Doping in Sport. Madrid, Spain (15 November).

Rose, A. L. and Everard, G. (2007). Injury prevention. *Coaching Edge*, 6, 24–5.

Rowett, H. G. Q. (1999). *Basic Anatomy and Physiology* (4th edn). John Murray, London.

Sackett, R. S. (1934). The influence of symbolic rehearsal upon the retention of a maze habit. *The Journal of General Psychology*, 10, 376–95.

Sandrock, M. (2000). *Running Tough*. Human Kinetics, Champaign, IL.

SAQ® (2003). *International Diploma in Training Speed, Agility and Quickness: Resource File*. Speed, Agility and Quickness International, Melton Mowbray, England.

SAQ® (2008). Online: http://www.saqinternational.com (accessed 28 September 2009).

Sawka, M. N., Burke, L. M., Eichner, E. R., Maughan, R. J., Montain, S. J. and Stachenfield, N. S. (2007). American College of Sports Medicine Position Stand on exercise and fluid replacement. *Medicine & Science in Sports & Exercise*, 39, 377–90.

Scarth, M., Foreman, G., Parsons, J. and Cruice, E. (2008). *Raising the Quality of Coaching: The UK Coaching Framework*. 3rd UK Coaching Summit, Coventry, 22–3 April.

Schmidt, R. A. (1975). A schema theory of discrete motor skill learning. *Psychological Review*, 82, 225–60.

Schmidt, R. A. (1991). *Motor Learning and Performance: From Principles to Practice*. Human Kinetics. Champaign, IL.

Schmidt, R. A. and Lee, T. (1999). *Motor Control and Learning: A Behavioural Emphasis*. Human Kinetics, Champaign, IL.

Schmidt, R. A. and Wrisberg, C. A. (2000). *Motor Learning and Performance: A Problem Based Learning Approach*. Human Kinetics, Champaign, IL.

Sellwood, K. C., Brukner, P., William, D., Nicol, A. and Hinman, R. (2007). Ice water immersion and delayed onset of muscle soreness: A randomized controlled trial. *British Journal of Sports Medicine*, 41, 392–7.

Shea, J. B. and Morgan, R. L. (1979). Contextual interference effects on the acquisition, retention and transfer of a motor skill. *Journal of Experimental Psychology: Human Learning and Memory*, 5, 179–87.

Sheik, A. A. and Korn, E. R. (1994). *Imagery in Sport and Physical Performance*. Baywood Publishing Company New York.

Shepherd, J. (2006). *The Complete Guide to Sports Training*. A & C Black, London.

Shrier, I. (1999). Stretching before exercise does not reduce the risk of local muscle injury: A critical review of the clinical and basic science literature. *Clinical Journal of Sports Medicine*, 9, 221–7.

SIA (2009). Self Improvement Association. Qualities of a true leader. Online: http://www.sia-hq.com/articles/14-Qualities-of-a-True-Leader (accessed 15th October 2009).

Siff, M. C. (2003). *Super Training* (6th edn). Super Training Institute, Denver, Colorado.

Smith, C. (2008). The cold benefits of ice baths. Online: http://news.bbc.co.uk/sportacademy/hi/sa/treatment_room/features/newsid_3097000/3097114.stm (accessed 28 September 2009).

Smith, R. E., Smoll, F. and Curtis, B. (1978). Coaching behaviours in little league baseball. In: R. E. Smith and F. Smoll (eds). *Psychological Perspectives in Youth Sport* (pp. 173–201). John Wiley & Sons, Toronto.

Smith, R. E., Smoll, F. L. and Hunt, E. (1977). A system of the behavioural assessment of athletic coaches. *The Research Quarterly*, 48(2), 401–7.

Smith-Nash, S. (2005). Goal-setting and self-regulation in online courses: The basics. Online: http://elearnqueen.blogspot.com/2005/12/goal-setting-and-self-regulation-in.html

SPARC (Sport and Recreation New Zealand), (2004). The New Zealand Coaching Strategy: Taking Coaching into the Future. Online: http://www.sparc.org.nz/sport/nz-coaching-strategy (accessed 28 September 2009).

Special Olympics (2007). Planning an Athletics Training and Competition Season. Special Olympics Athletics Coaching Guide. Online: http://info.specialolympics.org/Special+Olympics+Public+Website/English/Coach/Coaching_Guides/Athletics/Planning+a+Training+Season/default.htm (accessed 28 September 2009).

Spielberger, C. D. (1971). Trait-state anxiety and motor behaviour. *Journal of Motor Behaviour*, 3, 265–79.

Sport England (2002). About Clubmark. Online: http://www.clubmark.org.uk/about/about-clubmark (accessed 28 September 2009).

Sport England (2003). *Sports Volunteering in England 2002*. Sport England, London.

Sport England (2008). Online: http://www.sportengland.org (accessed 28 September 2009).

Sport Scotland (2003). *Ethics in Sport*. Caledonia House, South Gyle, Edinburgh.

SportsCoachUK (2001). *Code of Conduct for Sports Coaches*. SportsCoachUK, Leeds.

SportsCoachUK (2006). On the pulse: Cutting edge technology for coaches. *Coaching Edge*, 4.

SportsCoachUK (2007a). *The UK Coaching Framework: A 3–7–11 Year Action Plan*. SportsCoachUK, Leeds.

SportsCoachUK (2007b). Performance teams. *Coaching Edge*, 10(Winter).

SportsCoachUK (2008a). *History of SportsCoachUK*. SportsCoachUK, Leeds.

SportsCoachUK (2008b). *Coach Development Officers*. SportsCoachUK, Leeds.

SportsCoachUK (2008c). *UKCC Information*. SportsCoachUK, Leeds.

SportsCoachUK (2008d). *History of the UK Coaching Framework*. SportsCoachUK, Leeds.

SportsCoachUK (2008e). *Sports Coaching and the Law*. SportsCoachUK, Leeds.

SportsCoachUK (2008f). *Volunteer and Paid Coaching*. SportsCoachUK, Leeds.

SportsCoachUK (2008g). *Implications for Coaches of Impending Psychologists Legislation*. SportsCoachUK, Leeds.

SportsCoachUK (2008h). *License to Practice*. SportsCoachUK, Leeds.

SportsCoachUK (2008i). *Government Gives Green Light to Sports Skills Academy*. SportsCoachUK, Leeds.

SportsCoachUK (2008j). UK Vision for Coaching 2001: ch. 5. In: B. Taylor and D. Garratt (eds). *The Professionalization of Sports Coaching in the UK: Issues and Conceptualization*. SportsCoachUK, Leeds.

SportsCoachUK (2008k). *Career in Coaching*. SportsCoachUK, Leeds.

SportsCoachUK (2008l). *The UK Coaching Framework in Detail*. SportsCoachUK, Leeds.

SportsCoachUK (2008m). *Mentoring Review*. SportsCoachUK, Leeds.

SportsCoachUK (2008n). Coaches' key role in medal success. In: *The 2007 World Class Athlete Survey* (UK Sport 2007). SportsCoachUK, Leeds.

Sports Council (1988). *Sports in the Community: Into the 90s: A Strategy for Sport 1988–1993*. Sports Council, London.

SSP (Sussex Sports Partnership) (2004). *Sussex Sports Partnership Child Protection Policy*. University of Brighton, England.

Stafford, I. (2005). *Coaching for Long-term Athlete Development: To Improve Participation and Performance in Sport*. Coachwise/SportsCoachUK, Leeds.

Still, M. (2003). Why mentoring? *Faster, Higher, Stronger*, 18, 6.

Starkes, J. L. and Ericsson, K. A. (2003). *Expert Performance in Sports: Advances in Research on Sport Expertise*. Human Kinetics, Champaign, IL.

Szalma, J. L. and Hancock, P. A. (2009). White Paper: On mental resources and performance under stress. Department of Psychology and the Institute for Simulation and Training, University of Central Florida, pp. 1–14

Tamburrini, C. and Tannsjo, T. (2005). *Genetic Technology and Sport*. Routledge, London.

Tanaka, H., Monahan, K. D. and Seals, D. R. (2001). Age-predicted maximum heart rate re-visited. *Journal of American College of Cardiology*. 37, 153–6.

Taranowski, H. (2008). The importance of good nutrition in sport and fitness. Online: http://articles.getacoder.com/The_Importance_of_Good_Nutrition_in_Sport_and_Fitness_1556536x1217574239.htm (accessed 28 September 2009).

The Stretching Institute (2008). Cool down: Recover faster, avoid injury. Online: http://www.thestretchinghandbook.com/archives/cool-down.php (accessed 28 September 2009).

Thomas, A. (2000). Managing conflict. *Faster, Higher, Stronger*, 9, 26–7.

Torkildsen, G. (2005). *Leisure and Recreation Management*. Routledge, London.

Tortora, G. J. and Grabowski, S. R. (1996). *Principles of Anatomy and Physiology*. HarperCollins, New York.

Townend, R. and North, J. (2007). *Sports Coaching in the UK II: Main Report 2007*. SportsCoachUK, Leeds.

Treisman, A. (1998). Feature binding, attention and object perception. *Philosophical Transactions of the Royal Society of London*, 353, 1295–306.

UKCC (United Kingdom Coaching Certificate) (2008). Qualifications. Online: http://www.sportscoachuk.org/index.php?PageID=3&sc=9&uid= (accessed 15th October 2009).

UK Sport (2007). Giants get chance to show potential. Online: http://www.uksport.gov.uk/news/giants_get_chance_to_show_potential/ (accessed 28 September 2009).

UK Sport (2008a). Elite Coach. Online: http://www.uksport.gov.uk/pages/elite_coach/ (accessed 28 September 2009).

UK Sport (2008b). Performance lifestyle. Online: http://www.uksport.gov.uk/pages/performance_lifestyle/ (accessed 28 September 2009).

UK Sport (2008c). History of drug free sport. Online: http://www.uksport.gov.uk/pages/history_of_drug_free_sport/ (accessed 28 September 2009).

UK Sport (2008d). Sporting giants unearth over fifty hopefuls for 2012. Online: http://www.uksport.gov.uk/news/sporting_giants_one_year_on/ (accessed 28 September 2009).

UK Sport (2008e). New goal for young footballers as Olympic opportunity beckons. Online: http://www.uksport.gov.uk/news/new_goal_for_young_footballers_as_olympic_opportunity_beckons/ (accessed 28 September 2009).

UK Sport (2008f). WADA: Sport showing a greater interest in gene doping. Online: http://www.uksport.gov.uk/news/wada_sport_showing_greater_interest_in_gene_doping/ (accessed 28 September 2009).

UK Sport (2009a). Drug results show over 7,500 test conducted by UK Sport in last year. Online: http://www.uksport.gov.uk/news/dfs_end_of_year_results/ (accessed 28 September 2009).

UK Sport (2009b). Forums provide update on UKAD progress. Online: http://www.uksport.gov.uk/news/forums_provide_update_on_ukad_progress/ (accessed 28 September 2009).

USOC (United States Olympic Committee) (2008). Coaching Ethics Code. Online: http://www.asiaing.com/united-states-olympic-committee-coaching-ethics-code.html (accessed 28 September 2009).

Vander, A., Sherman, J. and Luciano, D. (1998). *Human Physiology: The Mechanisms of Body Function* (7th edn). WCB McGraw-Hill, New York.

Vallerand, R. J. (2001). A hierarchical model of intrinsic and extrinsic motivation in sport and exercise. In: G. C. Roberts (ed.). *Advances in Motivation in Sport and Exercise* (pp. 263–319). Human Kinetics, Champaign, IL.

Vealey, R. S. (1986). Conceptualization of sport-confidence and competitive orientation. Preliminary investigation and instrument development. *Journal of Sport Psychology*, 8, 221–46.

Venuto, T. (2009). Functional strength training vs bodybuilding: Is bodybuilding the worst thing that ever happened to strength training? Shawn Le Brawn Fitness. Online: http://www.shawnlebrunfitness.com/build-muscle/bodybuilding.html (accessed 28 September 2009).

Vygotsky, L. S. (1978). *Mind and Society: The Development of Higher Mental Processes*. Harvard University Press, Cambridge, MA.

WADA (2005). Gene doping. *Play True*, 1, 2–21.

Wadler, G. and Hainline, B. (1989). *Drugs and the Athlete*. Davis Publishing, Philadelphia.

Watkins, R. (1997). *Gladiators*. Houghton Mifflin Company, New York.

Watt, D. C. (2003). *Sports Management and Administration* (2nd edn). Routledge, London.

Weinberg, R. S. and Gould, D. (1999). *Foundations of Sport and Exercise Psychology*. (2nd edn). Human Kinetics, Champaign, IL.

Weinberg, R. S. and Gould, D. (2006). *Foundations of Sport and Exercise Psychology* (3rd edn). Human Kinetics, Champaign, IL.

Weinberg, R. S. and Gould, D. (2007). *Foundations of Sport and Exercise Psychology* (4th edn). Human Kinetics, Champaign, IL.

Weiss, M. R. (2004). Coaching children to embrace a "Love of the game". *USOC Olympic Coach*, 16(1), 15–17.

Welford, A. T. (1968). *Fundamentals of Skill*. Methuen, London.

Wertperch (2008). Jonny Wilkinson MBE. Online: http://www.everything2.com/index.pl?node=jonny+wilkinson&lastnode_id=124 (accessed 15th October 2009).

REFERENCES

Wilkinson, D. and Moore, P. (1995). *Measuring Performance: A Guide to Field Based Fitness Testing*. National Coaching Foundation, Leeds.

Williams, M. (2002). Perceptual and cognitive expertise in sport. *The Psychologist*, 15(8), 416–17.

Winstein, C. J. and Schmidt, R. A. (1990). Reduced frequency of knowledge of results enhances motor skill learning. *Journal of Experimental Psychology*, 15, 677–91.

Winstone, W. (2007). How much of a sport psychologist are you? *Coaching Edge*, 6, 20–1.

Winter, E. R. C., Jones, A. M., Davison, R., Bromley, P. and Mercer, T. (2006). *Sport and Exercise Physiology Testing Guidelines* (Vols I and II). Routledge, London.

Wirhead, R. (1984). *Athletic Ability and the Anatomy of Motion*. Moseby-Wolfe, London.

Wolstencroft, E. (2002). *Talent Identification and Development: An Academic Review*. Sport Scotland, Edinburgh.

Yates, I., Dunman, N. and Warr, C. (2007). Unearthing London 2012 talent: The latest in talent transfer. *Coaching Edge*, 9, 12–13.

Yerkes, R. M. and Dodson, J. D. (1908). The relation of strength stimulus to rapidity of habit formation. *Journal of Comparative Neurology and Psychology*, 18, 459–82.

Zaheen, A. (2008). A guide to Federer's playing style. Online: http://federermagic.blogspot.com/2005/03/guide-to-federers-playing-style.html (accessed 28 September 2009).

Zawadzki, K. M., Yaspelkis, B. B. III and Ivy, J. L. (1992). Carbohydrate protein complex increases the rate of muscle glycogen storage after exercise. *Journal of Applied Physiology*, 72(5), 1854–9.

Zbaracki, M.J. (1998). The rhetoric and reality of total quality management. *Administrative Science Quarterly*, 43(3), 602–36.

Zeigler, E. (1984). *Ethics and Morality in Sport and Physical Education: An Experimental Approach*. Stipes Publishing, Champaign, IL.

Zimmerman, B. J. and Kitsantas, A. (1996). Self regulated learning of a motoric skill: The role of goal setting and self monitoring. *Journal of Applied Sport Psychology*, 8, 69–84.

Index

Note: page numbers in **bold** refer to figures and tables.